"I enjoyed reading *The Neuroscience of Memory* because of the unique approach Sherrie All brings to the subject. She presents the elements of emotional intelligence with clarity and sound methodology that resonates with the work we do at the Wright Graduate University for the Realization of Human Potential. These down-to-earth, science-based tools provide so much more than the title implies—they are foundational to robust mental health and success in all aspects of life, from relationship to career."

—**Robert J. Wright, EdD**, award-winning, best-selling coauthor of
The Heart of the Fight and *Transformed!*

"Sooner or later, we all start worrying about our memories as we get older. In this book, Sherrie All provides an invaluable resource to help us assess our memories and maximize our potential. While she highlights relevant scientific findings, she also strikes a friendly and reassuring tone. Highly recommended for anyone who wants to make the best use of their brain in middle age or above!"

—**Jan Willer, PhD**, author of *The Beginning Psychotherapist's Companion* and
Could It Be Adult ADHD?

"As a professional who is passionate about delivering integrative content in life-changing, practical skills, I'm excited about Sherrie All's workbook, *The Neuroscience of Memory*. Much more than sound, evidence-based professional advice, All's warm, compassionate voice accompanies you like a caring and wise friend as you come to understand your brain and improve your memory through accessible exercises. Her helpful tools are delivered with straight talk, sensitivity, and encouragement."

—**Judith Wright, EdD**, cofounder and president of the Wright Graduate University
for the Realization of Human Potential; and award-winning, best-selling coauthor of
The Heart of the Fight and *Transformed!*

"In this incredibly helpful book, Sherrie All makes neuroscience simple by explaining brain health in a way that is clear and understandable. With humor, compassion, and tremendous expertise, she'll help you move from feeling afraid and helpless about your memory and cognitive functioning to hopeful and empowered. Her tools and tips are user-friendly and effective. We are living through a global stress epidemic and could all benefit from this book."

—**Joyce Marter, LCPC**, licensed psychotherapist, founder of Urban Bal
national public speaker, and author of *The Financial Mindset Fix*

"Sherrie All has drawn upon her extensive knowledge of neuroscience and decades of clinical experience to create a uniquely holistic and practical workbook that explains why cognition fails, how to strengthen cognition while managing the emotional reaction to cognitive decline, and, perhaps most important, how to prevent future cognitive failure. For many people, this book will be an essential guide to preserving cognitive ability across the lifespan."

>—**Anthony Y. Stringer, PhD, ABPP/CN**, professor and director of rehabilitation neuropsychology at Emory University

"Sherrie All makes neuroscience accessible and entertaining, and her workbook is packed with strategies for improving brain function. This is an incredible resource for anyone who wants to take charge of their memory and brain health."

>—**Sara Dittoe Barrett, PhD**, licensed clinical psychologist, owner and director of Cognitive Behavioral Associates of Chicago, and author of *The 4-Week Insomnia Workbook*

"Based on her long clinical experience and with a deep foundation in neuroscience, Sherrie All has ably developed an achievable, practical program empowering every aging individual determined to maintain and strengthen their most valuable possession—the brain. If you want to buttress your ability to make and keep cherished memories, this book is for you."

>—**Paul E. Bendheim, MD**, clinical professor of neurology at the University of Arizona College of Medicine, founder and chief medical officer at BrainSavers®, and author of *The Brain Training Revolution*

"*You* can improve how *your* brain works, and you can do things *now* to keep it working well in the future. That is the powerful message in this new book by Sherrie All. The user-friendly program described in this book gives you the power to make the right neuroscience-informed lifestyle adjustments to think better, feel better, and live better. Start now. Be here later. Enjoy and remember the journey more."

>—**Steven M. Silverstein**, professor of psychiatry, neuroscience, and ophthalmology at the University of Rochester Medical Center; and director of the Center for Retina and Brain

The
Neuroscience
of Memory

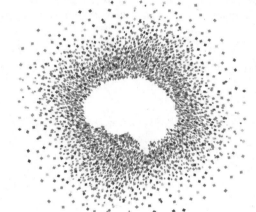

7 Skills to Optimize Your Brain Power,
Improve Memory, and Stay Sharp at Any Age

SHERRIE D. ALL, PhD

New Harbinger Publications, Inc.

Publisher's Note

Library of Congress Cataloging-in-Publication Data

Names: All, Sherrie, author. | Bendheim, Paul E., author.
Title: The neuroscience of memory : seven skills to optimize your brain power, improve memory, and stay sharp at any age / Sherrie All, Paul Bendheim.
Description: Oakland : New Harbinger Publications, 2021. | Includes bibliographical references.
Identifiers: LCCN 2020056043 | ISBN 9781684037438 (trade paperback)
Subjects: LCSH: Mental efficiency--Popular works. | Brain--Aging--Prevention--Popular works. | Self-help techniques--Popular works.
Classification: LCC BF431 .A553 2021 | DDC 153.9--dc23
LC record available at https://lccn.loc.gov/2020056043

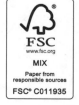
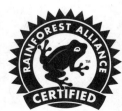

Printed in the United States of America

23   22   21

10   9   8   7   6   5   4   3   2   1

First Printing

To Ella, Lily, Charlie, and Alex. May you never be afraid to be badass women scientists or whatever you want to be.

Contents

Foreword

Of all the things I've lost, I miss my mind the most. —Mark Twain

You will never know the value of a moment, until it becomes a memory. —Dr. Seuss

We have just reached a unique juncture in the US, where for the first time, the number of people over the age of sixty-five has surpassed the number under the age of five. As our population ages, the fear of losing one's mind—losing one's memory—has become a leading health concern. Survey after survey documents this concern, and it is valid. We are currently in the initial phase of an epidemic of Alzheimer's disease, the leading cause of progressive dementia.

Every day ten thousand baby boomers turn sixty-five years old. Advancing age and unhealthy lifestyle practices are the two major risk factors for Alzheimer's disease. There were about six million people living with Alzheimer's disease in 2021, which will increase to fifteen million in the next thirty years—if we don't implement strategies to change this trajectory.

The above statistics sound grim and, until relatively recently, a grim prognosis was thought to be unavoidable. When I was a medical student and subsequently a neurology resident, the central dogma of the aging brain was that it was hardwired. When you reached the age of forty, this marvelous, hardwired computational organ—the seat of all distinguishing and unique human behavioral, emotional, thinking, learning, and creative functions—began to unravel. If you were fortunate, it unwound slowly; if you were unlucky, your brain unwound more rapidly, and you became demented (previously the term was "senile").

The good and encouraging news is that we have the ability to change this trajectory. As Dr. Sherrie All explains in the book you are holding, the neuroscience of the aging brain (what I have labeled "the new science of the aging brain") has at its core two principles: neuroplasticity and cognitive reserve. Neuroplasticity is the ability of your brain to change its anatomy, to create new brain cells and to connect them to other neurons. Cognitive (brain) reserve is the ability to build an insurance policy, a wall if you wish, against memory loss and the loss of other cognitive functions. Cognitive reserve diminishes the brain's wear and tear associated with normal aging (fewer memory misfires and senior moments), but most importantly, it reduces your risk of progressive cognitive decline resulting in Alzheimer's disease or vascular dementia.

Dr. All is a recognized neuropsychologist. She developed the Chicago Center for Cognitive Wellness and has helped countless patients dealing with the fear and the reality of memory loss. Her counseling and programs enrich lives while empowering individuals with the tools to improve memory formation, memory permanence, and memory recall. In this book, she not only explains the science behind the methodology for cognitive improvement and long-lasting brain health, but also asks hard questions of the reader to promote thinking and action about personal cognitive and memory issues. She then provides exercises and guidance, enabling the reader to better the brain both over the short term (working memory) and over the life span (long-term episodic and semantic memories).

To my personal satisfaction as a fervent advocate for a healthy brain lifestyle, Dr. All devotes separate chapters to the critically important components of lifestyle for aging individuals who want to enrich their lives while strengthening mind and body.

As is true with most endeavors in life, benefits come to those who work at it. Each of us has to be our own healthy brain quarterback. Fortunately, Dr. All's program, as elucidated in this volume, if initiated and committed to, will lead to real progress as you march up the field. As you experience the benefits while enjoying a richer, less stressful life, you will thank Dr. All for her leadership and easy-to-follow, evidence-based guidance.

—Paul E. Bendheim, MD

Clinical Professor of Neurology

University of Arizona College of Medicine–Phoenix

Author of *The Brain Training Revolution: A Proven Workout for Healthy Brain Aging*

Part I

Building Blocks

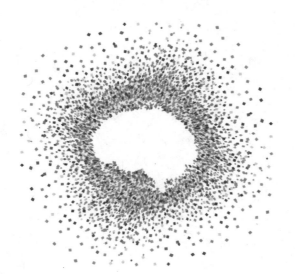

Introduction

Do you have a terrible memory? Would others agree, or do they say it's all in your head (pun intended)? Whether you legitimately have a terrible memory or not, I'm guessing by the fact that this book is in your hands you are concerned about your memory in some way. I imagine at the very least, you are curious, in search of answers, perhaps even frustrated. Maybe things are not what they used to be, or new challenges are arising.

It's Normal to Be Scared

Whether you've always had a terrible memory or are finding yourself slipping, you are not alone in your fear. Memory loss is a top fear (Kelley, Ulin, and McGuire 2018), and for good reason. Your fears are not frivolous. We rely heavily on our brains in our intelligence-based culture and economy. A sharp memory is a valuable resource; for many of us, it's the basis of our livelihoods, not to mention a source of pride and status. Take a moment to think about how much money it would cost you, in lost income, health care, and personal care expenses, if you had to stop working today or if people had to keep an eye on you because you kept leaving the stove on. Those numbers can quickly spiral up into the hundreds of thousands, and often millions, of dollars.

You may have already experienced some of these losses. If so, then you know all too well the impact that memory loss has on your bank account, not to mention your pride and your self-esteem. These changes can be devastating. Depression and anxiety are common and understandable reactions.

Worse than a loss of money, most people fear a loss of independence. What if you couldn't drive yourself places or set your own appointments? What if someone had put their life on hold to care for you? These scenarios aren't necessarily the end of the world. Increasingly this is becoming the reality for many as they care for aging parents. I mention it though to acknowledge the fear most people hold regarding what it would mean to lose memory skills. I'm also guessing that these are some of the deep, perhaps unnamed, fears that drove you to pick up this book.

No matter your circumstance, there is a lot you can do, so I'm glad you came here for help.

How to Use This Workbook

This is a workbook. Therefore, I have filled it with exercises and places to write your thoughts, goals, and plans. My intention is for you to use these activities to build a better memory. Some of the worksheets you might wish to print out or use again and again; therefore, many of the worksheets are available on the website for this book: http://newharbinger.com/47438.

The surveys are not diagnostic. They are here to help you better understand your individual brain and memory and to help you identify your strengths, which you will use to help support, bolster, and supplement your weaker areas. While I don't anticipate this being the case for everyone, some surveys may lead you to feel anxiety or raise your awareness of your memory to a point where you need to seek professional support. In such cases, please seek that support, and I encourage you to not shy away from the activities out of fear. Feeling fear is important; it can lead you to action. Plus, information is power, and help is available and transformative.

The exercises are designed for you to practice the skills I'm teaching you. In each chapter you will learn about a principle of neuroscience or a proven strategy for improved memory. You will then support your understanding and adoption of these principles and skills for lasting change through the exercises. You get out of them what you put into them.

The Long Game and the Need for Practice

Our journey together will likely take time—weeks, months, maybe even years—and that's okay. "Turtle speed" really is the rate of lasting change, whether we want to admit it or not. To really get the most out of this book, you should commit to a pattern of daily attention. Schedule in your calendar daily or weekly sessions with your workbook. You will be setting goals for yourself to practice the strategies I will teach you, often practicing each technique for a week at a time.

I'm not just making up this need for practice. What neuroscience and memory workbook would be complete without looking at what neuroscience has to say on the topic? Neuroscience tells us *repetition matters. Do the exercises.* Practice your new skills. This is because you are working to *rewire your brain* for a better memory. Rewiring doesn't happen in a flash. To develop better memory skills, you must practice them, repeat them, overlearn them, and maintain them, which means *repeat* them. To this end, I have structured many of the memory exercises in a way that will give you opportunities to practice them as you learn the neuroscience behind it all. This book is different than your standard memory trick book. You may find that many of the exercises seem to be more about neuroscience than memory. We are using neuroscience to help you improve your learning and memory. Building a better memory is all about learning better, and what better opportunity to practice learning than by learning? Many exercises are there to help you learn about neuroscience, and by using the strategies to learn and remember a new topic, you get to practice them in preparation to learn other topics. As you learn more about brain plasticity (this is the way the adult brain changes and remolds itself), the need for practice will become even clearer. Understanding neuroscience may not make you *want* to do the exercises any more than you do right now, but you will understand the neural basis of why practicing is so important.

Meet Cindy, Your Companion on This Journey

Cindy Williams is forty-seven years old. She has three kids, ages ten, thirteen, and seventeen. She works full time and shares custody with her ex-husband. Cindy enjoys her job but is often overwhelmed by office politics. About five years ago, Cindy sustained a concussion when someone at work opened the door to the break room too quickly, and the door smacked her in the head. She didn't lose consciousness, but she woke up the next day with a terrible headache and felt like garbage. This happened in the heat of her divorce. She tried to not take time off work at first, but after weeks of headaches, dizziness, brain fog, and tiredness, she finally met with HR to start a worker's compensation claim, which allowed her to take some time off.

At first doctors seemed to dismiss her fears and concerns, trying to be upbeat about her prognosis. She felt invalided, as though people thought she was making it all up and she was lazy. She finally found a good therapist, one she liked, and a good rehab and pain doctor, but she felt as if the worker's compensation company was judging her and pushing her to go back to work before she was ready.

Ever since all of this happened, she consistently worries about her memory. She wonders, *Will I get Alzheimer's like my grandma?* Every time Cindy forgets an appointment, which happens every month or so, she beats herself up, feeling fearful and ashamed.

Cindy hasn't been sleeping well since the accident and the divorce. Besides, who sleeps well with teenagers anyway? She takes Tylenol PM every night to help with this. She and the kids live on a steady diet of takeout, because who has time to cook, let alone get to the gym? After getting home, organizing the kids, and filling everyone's bellies, the best she can do is plop on the couch for some *Grey's Anatomy* and Candy Crush with a glass of Chardonnay and the corked bottle nearby. She tells herself she's only going to have one glass, though that rarely works out. She wonders, *Is this all there is? Am I doomed to a life in the nursing home? Can't I do something to improve my memory?*

Her fingers wander away from Candy Crush and over to the Amazon app on her phone, the lifeblood of any mom these days. She finds this neuroscience and memory workbook and orders it. Like you, she starts working through the exercises, changing her life, changing her memory, and changing her brain.

It's My Pleasure to Be Your Guide

Throughout our journey together, I will be guiding you, and Cindy, through a deeper understanding of your brain, focusing on how it supports your memory. I will guide you through how it works and how it fails you. By developing a deeper understanding of how your brain works, you will be equipped with more tools to operate it better.

I have been helping people improve their thinking for nearly two decades. I am excited and honored to have the opportunity to support you on your journey of memory improvement, and I am grateful that you have invited me to accompany you along this journey.

Why Neuroscience? (Not Just Another Memory Book)

Over the last two decades, the field of neuroscience has been turned upside down by new research showing that the adult brain can and does change in positive ways throughout the entire life span, molding itself based on how we use it. This new science has, in turn, dramatically changed the way we understand memory and the approaches needed to maximize its function. Drawing on the latest neuroscience to help you avoid futility in your memory-enhancement efforts, I will guide you in understanding the latest evidence about how your brain works, which will help you effectively guide your efforts toward your personal memory goals.

You will learn how your physical state can enhance or impair your memory, providing you the motivation you need to eat your veggies, get plenty of sleep, and move your body, like the experts say to do. You will learn the biology behind why moments of intense emotion can either highlight or hijack your memories. This knowledge will give you control. You will also learn and practice tried-and-true memory techniques, all while learning how to best operate the organ running the show.

Meta-Cognition

The neuro (brain) plus the science elements of this book are useful because when you know how your memory actually works inside your brain, you are better equipped to use it. Research in the field of cognitive rehabilitation—a set of evidence-based interventions to improve memory and other cognitive skills, such as attention in people who have experienced a decline due to injury or disease—has shown that when people understand how the brain works, they are better able to control and improve its function. This "meta-cognitive" approach (which means "thinking about thinking") results in the best outcomes for patients when these rehabilitation interventions are put to the test (Cicerone et al. 2011). Interventions that do not include this type of neuroscience-informed education result in weaker outcomes.

Take charge of your memory. Enhancing your memory with neuroscience puts you in the driver's seat to change and grow your brain and memory. So let's get started.

Chapter 1

The Gifts of Neuroscience

Maybe you've always had a terrible memory; maybe you haven't. Maybe you recently sustained a concussion or just went through chemo. There is no faster way to become incredibly aware of memory glitches than to experience a period when your brain just doesn't work like it used to. (Ahem, pregnancy and sleepless nights with a newborn anyone?) Maybe you've been diagnosed with MS or Parkinson's disease or you got bit by that ill-fated tick and contracted Lyme disease. Now you are left wondering, *What's in store for me if I lose my memory skills?* Maybe you're feeling your old bones and noticing the changes that come naturally with age, but understandably this has you worried. Like many of the people who visit my office, you likely feel scared. At the very least, I'm sure it's safe to say that you are not satisfied with your memory, and you are looking for solutions.

Why Do You Want to Improve Your Memory?

Take a moment to journal about why you picked up this book. This will help you acknowledge some of your fears and set the stage for addressing them as we work together.

_____

_____

_____

_____

_____

_____

_____

What did you put down? Do you want a better memory to show off or compete in memory competitions? I'm guessing probably not. I'll bet you listed reasons related to wanting to be better at your job or a more attentive parent, grandparent, partner, or friend. You might also be fearing the dark cloud of dementia looming on the horizon and want to remain as independent and productive as long as possible. I'm betting that you want evidence-based strategies that will keep your brain strong and vibrant, not parlor tricks.

That's what I want for you, and using a neuroscience approach is the best way to get you there. Advances in neuroscience over the last twenty years have revealed many surprises, leading us to reprioritize what we recommend for memory-enhancement strategies. This new science will help you focus your efforts in a way that will be most effective in helping you meet the "why" and intentions you listed above. Many adult brains are getting bigger throughout the life span. Did you know that? However, many are getting smaller. Which group will you be in?

Is It All in My Head?

Since I'm not your doctor, I have no way of knowing if your memory concerns are clinical concerns or not. It could very well be the case that something is wrong with your memory and your underlying brain. On the other hand, your brain may be just fine. Or, you may not be worried at all, and you picked up this book to just give yourself an edge. All great starting points.

If you are worried about your brain, the only real way to know if your struggles are normal or not is to get your brain checked out by a doctor. I'm a big advocate of getting all of that checked out, which typically involves consulting with a couple of different doctors. You'll need your medical doctor to order blood tests and a brain scan. Some primary care physicians do this, but many will refer you to a neurologist. A neurologist can quickly screen for memory changes and will know whether your memory is okay or not, but in many cases, the neurologist's test is not sensitive enough. The gold standard for a dementia diagnosis is formal neuropsychological testing by a clinical neuropsychologist, with insurance covering this service in most cases.

Neuropsychological testing is sort of like IQ testing but broader, testing all brain skills, including memory. You sit down with a trained professional for about three to six hours and work through a variety of tasks. Most are interactive or paper and pencil based. Some of the tests are on a computer, but be wary of offers to do the entire assessment on a computer as there can be serious validity issues with these types of tests.

I'm passionate about neuropsychological assessment, and not just because it's my professional background and a foundational offering in my clinic. In almost every case, objective testing of your memory is the only way to really know if something is wrong or if you're worried about it for no reason. It is a really good idea to have a professional weigh in on which cognitive skills you may be losing, how much your skills are or are not slipping, and what they think is the cause, because guess what? You can do something about it!

Maybe you already knew this or were hopeful, otherwise why would you be reading this book, right? My point is that a lot of people avoid testing out of the fear that it will provide useless knowledge: "Why bother knowing if I have a memory problem if I can't do anything about it?" You can do something about it, and a formal assessment will give you an idea of what to do both in terms of how concerned you need to be or not and where to focus your efforts.

Collect your thoughts. Jot down some of your thoughts at this moment. List some of your fears. Do you want to see a doctor? What might you ask?

The Delicate and Resilient Human Brain

It's awe-inspiring that our brains work as well as they do given the number of things that can go wrong. Have you ever had that feeling of awe when you consider, *How does this all come together and actually work?* Merriam-Webster defines "awe" as "an emotion variously combining dread, veneration, and wonder that is inspired by authority or by the sacred or sublime." You may have felt this when you held a newborn baby or visited a national park. That's how I feel about the brain. The very fact that this organ comes together in the first twenty-eight days after conception, has more cells at birth than it will ever have again, is almost fully formed by age twenty-five, and in most cases does this flawlessly is simply amazing and awe-inspiring.

A big reason why the brain is so awesome is because it is equally powerful and delicate, just like life itself. In light of the number of things that can go wrong with your brain, it is amazing how this three-pound mass of goo—so fragile it has to sit deep inside a dense skull, suspended in liquid so it doesn't bruise itself—more often than not develops itself into a complicated, self-correcting super-computer more powerful than any computer ever built or even imagined.

Your brain, made up of billions of cells and trillions of connections, is more sophisticated than an iPhone, and I know, that thing is amazing, right? These days I'm convinced my phone knows more about me than I do, but guess what? Your brain is smarter than that phone. Smartphones are sophisticated because of all the different networks they synthesize. Your brain synthesizes networks, too, except better than artificial intelligence.

Often, we take all of this power for granted, and then we get upset when our brains don't work the way we want. We scratch our heads or call ourselves dumb when we are foggy the morning after a night of heavy drinking, taking a Benadryl, or not getting enough sleep. Add to that an underfunctioning heart, fluctuations in blood sugar from diabetes, or any other of a plethora of physical ailments that can leave you not feeling so sharp, and it is no wonder we worry about our memory.

Your brain is delicate because it depends on basically every organ system in your body to keep its cells alive and functioning properly. When something goes wrong in your body (heart, lungs, kidneys, liver, and so forth), it can dramatically impact your brain. Some physical issues are temporary, but others can be more permanent.

Collect your thoughts. Jot down some thoughts as you consider the brain as a delicate organ subject to lots of interference.

_____

_____

_____

_____

But Don't Get Too Freaked Out

It is important to not go overboard with concern over what's damaging your memory. Most of the time our brains are just fine. For a physical problem to affect your brain function in a way that is detectible on neuropsychological testing, it is typically a rather big event. Therefore, I encourage you to assume the best.

If you do fear the worst, though, please put down this book right now and pick up the phone to make an appointment with your doctor. Do it now. It really can't hurt to get a checkup. You don't have to wait six months to get in with a neurologist either. Go see your primary care physician. They can take your blood pressure, measure your B_{12} level, and ask you questions about how bad it is.

What Have You Seen or Heard?
What Are Your Thoughts About Memory Loss?

It is a good idea to be honest with yourself about what biases you have about memory loss that may be driving any anxiety or fear. List people you've watched or are watching struggle with memory loss or other cognitive changes. (I've included a couple of Cindy's fears to help you get started.)

Person	Your Thoughts and Feelings About This
Grandma Sue	It was just so sad when she couldn't remember who we were. My mom was so stressed-out. I don't want to be a burden on my kids, and it will be so embarrassing to not remember their names.

Great job. Understanding your fears and biases is really important as you work toward improving your memory because fear and judgment are profound barriers to memory performance. I want you to get a good sense of your biases about memory loss and dementia to clear the way for you to engage more fully in your work to improve your memory.

Your Personal Problem

I can't diagnose your personal problem unless you are in my clinic, so we will need to paint broad strokes. Memory loss comes in many forms, from many different sources, but the main sources are problems caused by a disease like Alzheimer's or Parkinson's, an injury from a blow to the head, or an internal injury from a stroke. Problems can also arise from things going wrong in the body like a heart, lung, or kidney problem. Memory also changes naturally with age and life circumstances, and people also vary greatly in their individual strengths and weaknesses.

I have a friend who describes herself as having a very terrible memory, but I really don't think that's true. I haven't had the chance to test her memory yet, but she describes herself as someone who never remembers what people tell her. Through further conversation, though, I learned that she uses a lot of strategies to remember information visually, drawing mental pictures of things that people tell her. I see this as a strength, and I doubt her memory is as terrible as she thinks because she is very successful, juggling lots of responsibilities. But because she has a narrow view of memory, expecting herself to remember what she hears and discounting her visualization strategy, she spends a lot of time worrying, I believe, unnecessarily.

Now is a good time to inventory the specific problems you are having with your memory and other thinking skills.

Memory Complaint Checklist

Check all the cognitive symptoms on the list below that apply to you currently. "Onset" refers to when you first noticed the problem. Have you had it all your life, or is it new? Write the age you were when you noticed the problem. You don't have to be precise. There is also room for you to describe your specific experiences. My clinic sends this checklist to all of our patients before they come in for a neuropsychological assessment. Completing it can help you prepare for seeing a neuropsychologist or a neurologist. You can download this form at http://newharbinger.com/47438 to print and take with you to doctor's appointments if you don't want to lug this whole book around.

Symptom	Onset	Describe (for those checked)
☐ Short-term memory problems		
☐ Asking repetitive questions		
☐ Forgetting details of conversations		
☐ Forgetting appointments		

☐ Misplacing items		
☐ Forgetting to take medications		
☐ Word-finding problems		
☐ Spelling, reading, or writing difficulty		
☐ Problems with calculations		
☐ Getting lost in familiar places		
☐ Problems paying attention		
☐ Distractibility		
☐ Disorganization		
☐ Problems planning or organizing		
☐ Difficulty following through/ finishing tasks		
☐ Personality changes		

Additional cognitive symptoms (changes in your thinking skills not listed above):

_____

_____

_____

_____

_____

Having one, three, or even five or more of the symptoms above does not guarantee that something terrible is happening to your brain. The Alzheimer's Association provides a handy guide called "Know the 10 Signs," which you can complete in the next chapter.

Society's Problem

We are facing a major public health crisis in most post-WWII industrialized countries. The prevalence of dementia, driven in large part by the ever-dreaded Alzheimer's disease, is expected to triple in the next thirty years unless preventative measures are developed (Herbert et al. 2013). Why is this trend happening?

People are living longer, but that's been happening for a long time. The source of the current crisis is that ten thousand baby boomers turn sixty-five every single day in the United States, a trend that has been happening for nearly a decade at the writing of this book and is expected to continue for nearly another decade. And what is the number one risk factor for dementia? Being over age sixty-five.

The social and economic impact of this crisis is startling and sobering. The projected costs to the United States in 2050 from just Alzheimer's disease, not to mention stroke and other dementias, are expected to top $1 trillion per year. Health care costs are only the tip of the iceberg. Eighty-five percent of the cost of dementia comes from nonmedical sources, including lost wages and expensive personal care (Livingston et al. 2017). The *Lancet Commissions* published a review in 2017 that described dementia as "the greatest global challenge for health and social care in the twenty-first century" (Livingston et al. 2017, 3). (This was reported before the 2020 pandemic, so it may not be currently true. But still a big deal.)

The Problem for Anyone Over Twenty-Five

Even if you don't have dementia or aren't even close, you may be noticing the declines in memory that occur naturally with age. For younger adults, these changes can be subtle, and you may chalk it up to changes in your lifestyle, which are real, such as being a new parent or the learning curve in starting a new job. As you get a little further over the hill, those "excuses" become a little harder to accept. *Why can't I learn this new app? Why is it so hard to remember my new address? I used to be so good at this stuff.* Well, that is actually true. I'm sorry to say. You probably *were* better at remembering things when you were twenty. It's a sobering fact.

The sad reality is that except for a couple of cognitive skills—like your vocabulary and your wisdom, both of which continue to improve throughout the life span—*every other cognitive skill peaks at around age twenty-five and steadily declines from there* (Salthouse 2009). I'm sorry. It is depressing to realize this, especially if you are locked in a battle of wills with a young adult child who is convinced they have grown smarter than you, because, truth be told, in many ways they are now (they're quicker at learning than you but definitely not wiser). On the other hand, like most things related to "adulting," admitting and accepting this "over-twenty-five" reality can help you (1) interrupt any fear and shame spirals that you might go into when you can't remember something and (2) take control of the process, which is the purpose of this book.

Just because these skills decline naturally with age doesn't mean there is *nothing* you can do about it. Your brain can still adapt and improve. That means your memory skills can also adapt and improve. It is unlikely that you are going to be able to train yourself to kick your fifteen-year-old's butt in the game called "who can text dad to buy more milk the fastest." (Go ahead and outsource that stuff anyway. Why else did you have the kid in the first place?) You can adopt strategies for remembering things in your everyday life in a way that will help you continue to kick butt at life, and I'm here to help you do that.

Neuroscience Offers a New Source of Hope

We used to think that the adult brain was fixed and hardwired, but we now know this is not the case. There is much more hope now than the neuroscience community would have offered you twenty, fifteen, or even ten years ago. We now have solid evidence that proves that you can change your brain and improve your thinking skills across your entire lifetime.

Hope comes in many forms. It can come in the form of understanding and compassion. It can also come in the form of solutions. This workbook is filled with both. Many solutions are practical strategies for improving memory, while others are attitude based, like challenging self-defeating thoughts and beliefs. Regardless of the severity of your memory problems at this very moment, a lot can shift for you in terms of how you tackle your life; gain, maintain, and sustain independence; and most importantly, improve your memory performance.

Tempered Hope

How much memory improves will vary from person to person, injury to injury, and so forth. If you have experienced moderate to severe cognitive declines, you will likely have to temper some expectations. You may not be able to improve your actual memory abilities, per se. The focus will be more on ways to compensate for your memory or attention declines. I never want to be Pollyannaish when trying to instill hope around memory improvements; this rehab stuff can be really hard. If cognition can't or won't improve, other things like daily functioning, independence, and mood can improve. Your current reality doesn't have to be your permanent reality. A lot can shift for you depending on how you react to your circumstances, sometimes through improving memory function and other times through compensation or a shift in perspective.

Everyone needs to temper expectations on some level. Be wary of products and programs that claim that your memory scores will jump up after some intervention or pill, especially claims that will "raise your IQ." Cognitive and IQ scores simply do not jump up.

Hope Through Vision

Draw a picture of yourself celebrating your start on your path to a better memory—it can be as simple as an emoji or as detailed as you sitting on the beach at sunset or hitting the piñata at your hopefulness party. You might find this exercise silly, but as you will find in this book, visualization is a key memory strategy, so let's get you started on it now. While you're at it, draw a vision of yourself with a sharper memory.

Me Celebrating My Start	Me in the Future with a Better Memory

Is This the Right Book for Me?

Whatever your reason for picking up this book, from sharpening your skills to overcoming a decline to warding off Alzheimer's, you have come to the right place. The promise of neuroscience is here to help you, and I'm here to do what I love best, which is to teach you about neuroscience in what I hope is a fun and relatable way.

Why learn about neuroscience? Knowing about neuroscience will help you more effectively guide your efforts as you work to improve your memory skills and change your life. Throughout this book, I will teach you how memory works in your brain, highlighting the myriad of ways it can and will go awry, and guide you in getting things on track. I will share with you my hopefulness for your memory and help you understand the realities of your brain, along with the innovations of the past twenty years that have, like never before, expanded the optimism for memory improvements. My goal is to help you use this information as a guide and a motivator as you practice new behaviors that are proven to improve memory in everyday life.

I believe that this book is useful for anyone wishing to improve their memory. That said, I particularly intend to reach four main groups of people. These are the people my staff and I work with daily. They include:

1. Adults or adolescents who have experienced a sudden and/or drastic decline in thinking skills due to illness or injury, including concussion, traumatic brain injury (TBI), stroke, or dementia.

2. Adults noticing slow changes in their thinking who are afraid that they are starting on the path to dementia.

3. People with complicated lives, often with high-powered jobs and/or demanding family situations, who sense that their brains could work more effectively, but who also feel frustrated and therefore want proven techniques to achieve this.

4. People who panic nearly every time they forget something but have been told there doesn't seem to be any medical reason to support their concerns.

People in all four categories show up to our office at every age. Those over fifty are typically convinced they're getting dementia; those under fifty have often experienced a concussion or fear they have ADHD. Whatever your reason for picking up this book, I believe you're in the right place. My aim is to help you understand your brain so you can best guide its function no matter what's going on under the hood.

So now that you know this is the right book for you, and you know how to work the workbook, let's get started.

Chapter 2

Why People Have Memory Problems

It's clear you want more from your memory, so now let's dig into why you may be struggling with your memory. In this chapter, you will learn that not all roads lead to the nursing home. I will start by helping you get a sense of the many causes of memory loss, and then I will describe some broad categories that people with memory complaints fall into.

This chapter is peppered with self-assessments to help you get a better sense of your memory challenges and help you focus on the possible discussions that you may have with your doctor. You will also practice your first memory skill.

Get More Accurate About Your Memory

Memory is impacted by a plethora of physical, emotional, and behavioral factors. Most factors are benign and addressable. My aim is to prove to you (via neuroscience) that you can struggle with your memory for a variety of reasons, not because you're stupid or you're deep in the throes of dementia. I'm emphasizing this because I know how often people jump to these conclusions; I hear these fears on a daily basis.

My goal is to remove the phrase "my memory sucks" from your vocabulary and replace it with something more accurate, such as (1) "I didn't pay close enough attention to what you said," (2) "I'm feeling really anxious right now and can't concentrate," or (3) "My doctor says the part of my brain responsible for my memory recall is impaired. I can still learn things; I just need to take some notes to reference later."

What Causes Memory Problems?

Many things cause memory problems. If we were to discuss all the causes of memory loss, it would take us about three to four years. Neurologists and neuropsychologists spend years studying these causes so they can tell you what's affecting your individual memory. I can't tell you what's causing your memory problems, but what I can do is provide you with an overview of the common causes of memory loss. The checklist below will help you get a sense of the many things that can affect memory as you start to assess what might be at the root of your personal memory challenges.

It's Not Always Dementia

It is not accurate to think of the list below as "causes of dementia," but rather "things that can affect memory." "Dementia," or what we are now calling "major neurocognitive disorder" (major NCD), is defined as a significant decline in at least one cognitive skill (these include memory; attention; executive functions, which are skills like planning and organizing; language; visual and spatial skills—basically how your brain processes visual information; and social skills, including empathy and personality) that is worse than that which occurs with normal aging, keeps you from being independent, isn't temporary (like a vitamin deficiency or delirium), and isn't caused by another mental disorder, like depression (American Psychiatric Association 2013). The difference between dementia and Alzheimer's disease is that dementia is the syndrome of cognitive skill loss (the symptoms) that I just described, not a disease. Alzheimer's is a disease that grows in the brain and causes the dementia syndrome. Lots of other things cause dementia or major NCD, such as stroke, traumatic brain injury (TBI), and Parkinson's disease.

There are many conditions beyond the much-dreaded progressive Alzheimer's disease that cause memory changes, and most conditions have a better prognosis. Be wary of programs that tout their ability to "reverse Alzheimer's disease," because, as of the writing of this book, we can't do that yet. The success stories touted in those programs typically involve correcting a chemical imbalance or vitamin deficiency that we never would have called dementia or Alzheimer's in the first place. I'll elaborate on a couple of these categories later. In the meantime, spend some time evaluating your personal history on the checklist below to get a better sense of your risk factors for memory loss.

Common Causes of Memory Complaints Checklist

(You can download a printable copy of this checklist at http://newharbinger.com/47438 in case you want to have it handy to take to your doctor at some point.)

Brain diseases (Most of these are not things you are going to know you have unless someone like a neurologist has told you so.):

- ☐ Alzheimer's disease
- ☐ Parkinson's disease
- ☐ Huntington's disease
- ☐ Lewy body dementia
- ☐ Frontotemporal dementia
- ☐ Pick's disease

Infections:

- ☐ Viruses or bacteria that enter the brain (this is called encephalitis)
- ☐ Viruses or bacteria that enter the outer coverings of the brain and spinal cord (called meningitis)
- ☐ Human immunodeficiency virus (HIV)
- ☐ Creutzfeldt-Jakob's disease or prion disease (the human form of mad cow disease)

Injury:

- ☐ A blow to the head causing a loss of consciousness
- ☐ A blow to the head that did not result in loss of consciousness but did result in concussion symptoms (headache, dizziness, balance problems, double vision, fatigue, mental confusion, irritability, and so forth)
- ☐ Brain surgery
- ☐ Stroke (a bleed in the brain or a blockage in blood flow)
- ☐ TIA (transient ischemic attack), or ministroke or silent stroke
- ☐ Anoxia or hypoxia (oxygen deprivation from a heart attack, carbon monoxide poisoning, and so forth)

Chemical- or substance-induced damage:

- ☐ Long-term damage from heavy alcohol use
- ☐ Long-term use of certain anxiety or sleep medications
- ☐ Heavy metal poisonings, for example from lead or mercury
- ☐ Long-term exposure to industrial solvents

Cardiac conditions:

- ☐ Heart disease
- ☐ Heart attack
- ☐ Congestive heart failure
- ☐ Atrial fibrillation (AFib)
- ☐ Any sort of cardiac valve dysfunction
- ☐ Cardiac bypass
- ☐ Blood clots
- ☐ Peripheral artery disease

Lung conditions:

- ☐ Chronic obstructive pulmonary disease (COPD)
- ☐ Asthma
- ☐ Lung cancers

Other organs:

- ☐ Kidney disease or damage
- ☐ Liver damage

Sensory loss:

- ☐ Uncorrected hearing loss
- ☐ Uncorrected vision loss
- ☐ Macular degeneration
- ☐ Cataracts

Delirium (a temporary decline in mental status caused by a physical issue):

- ☐ Medication toxicity caused by the wrong dose or medication interactions
- ☐ Urinary tract infection in older adults
- ☐ Mental confusion after anesthesia
- ☐ Sepsis
- ☐ Electrolyte imbalance or severe dehydration

Chronic diseases (These can cause excessive wear and tear on the brain and/or lower function periodically.):

- ☐ Diabetes
- ☐ Congestive heart failure
- ☐ Hypertension / high blood pressure

Brain mechanical failures:

- ☐ Epilepsy (faulty electrical wiring in the brain)
- ☐ Normal-pressure hydrocephalus (NPH, a clogged drainage system for spinal fluid in the brain)

Autoimmune disorders:

- ☐ Multiple sclerosis (MS)
- ☐ Lupus
- ☐ Sarcoidosis
- ☐ Hashimoto's disease / autoimmune limbic encephalopathy
- ☐ Thyroid dysfunction

Cancer:

- ☐ Brain tumors
- ☐ Fatigue and toxicity caused by chemo and radiation
- ☐ Brain disease related to cancer elsewhere in the body

Vitamin deficiencies:

- ☐ B_{12}
- ☐ Thiamine
- ☐ Omega-3s and antioxidants, which are important for long-term brain health

Medications and other substances:

- ☐ Steroids, such as Prednisone
- ☐ Beta blockers
- ☐ Benzodiazepines, such as Xanax and Klonopin
- ☐ Sedating antihistamines, such as Benadryl, NyQuil, Dramamine
- ☐ Over-the-counter sleep meds, such as Unisom or Tylenol PM
- ☐ Antipsychotic medications, such as Seroquel (quetiapine), Abilify, Haldol (haloperidol), Risperdal (risperidone), Thorazine
- ☐ Anticholinergic medications, such as Artane, that are used to reduce the motor side effects of some antipsychotics
- ☐ Some bipolar and epilepsy medications (older sedating ones, such as Topamax)
- ☐ Opiates
- ☐ Marijuana/THC
- ☐ Alcohol

Fatigue:

- ☐ Sleep apnea
- ☐ Sleep disorders
- ☐ Insomnia
- ☐ Periodic limb movement disorder (PLMD)
- ☐ Restless legs syndrome (RLS)
- ☐ Life, stress, toddlers, and so forth
- ☐ Chronic fatigue / Epstein-Barr virus

Emotions:

- ☐ Anxiety
- ☐ Trauma
- ☐ Depression
- ☐ Flooding (being overwhelmed with emotion)
- ☐ Freezing (becoming immobilized by stress, feeling faint)
- ☐ Dissociation (checking out mentally—lights are on, nobody's home; losing time)
- ☐ Psychosis (hearing voices, paranoia, and so forth)

Defeating beliefs:

- ☐ Believe it or not, believing your memory sucks can easily become a self-fulfilling prophecy (not that your memory is in the end organically damaged, but your daily performance suffers)

Pretty big list, right? Did you check off any of these? If you have any of the physical, medical, or emotional conditions listed above and they are not well controlled with the help of a physician or counselor, I strongly encourage you to seek professional support. Don't delay. As you will learn later on, many of the above physical, medical, and emotional conditions cause memory complaints now and are risk factors for dementia later on, so even if you don't think the impact is serious right now, it could spell big trouble later on.

The good news is that most, if not all, of the conditions above are treatable, and when treated, the impact on brain and memory can be remarkably reduced. Most physicians are keeping an eye on brain health these days, working with patients with long-term brain health in mind.

Four Main Types of Memory Problems

I find that many people believe that every form of memory loss is progressive, meaning it will get worse over time. Perhaps this is because of the high prevalence of Alzheimer's disease, which is progressive. The truth is that progressive dementias are only one type of memory loss. Many other causes of memory loss have a positive trajectory, meaning we actually expect people to get better over time, not worse

I'd like for you to think about memory problems in four main categories: (1) progressive conditions, like Alzheimer's disease, where the long-term course is downward; (2) static declines that occur after a stroke or brain injury where the initial memory loss is the most severe, but over time skills improve; (3) what I call "anxiety, trauma, and false beliefs," which takes some explaining, so keep reading; and (4) health conditions and lifestyle patterns that dull your skills.

1. Progressive Conditions

Let's be real. The biggest, scariest potential reality for most people is getting or already having a progressive dementia like Alzheimer's disease. I've known people who worry about this at virtually every stage of adulthood, but the fear definitely gets stronger as people get older. I don't blame you for being worried, particularly if you are creeping up on age sixty-five, or maybe you've blown way past it. Alzheimer's disease is the most common form of dementia, and the biggest risk factor for Alzheimer's disease is being over sixty-five. However, that does not mean that just because you're over sixty-five that you *will* get Alzheimer's disease.

To get a better sense of whether or not you are struggling with something progressive like Alzheimer's disease, the Alzheimer's Association (2009) has a handy worksheet called "Know the 10 Signs." This worksheet is a good place to log all of your worries and concerns, plus you can take this with you to doctors' appointments. In this way you will have logged your concerns ahead of time and will be all set to discuss them. If you find that you have symptoms on the list, I do recommend you call your doctor. *(You can access this form at http://newharbinger.com/47438.)*

Know the 10 Signs: Early Detection Matters

HAVE YOU NOTICED ANY OF THESE WARNING SIGNS?

Please list any concerns you have and take this sheet with you to the doctor.

Note: This list is for information only and not a substitute for a consultation with a qualified professional.

☐ **1. Memory loss that disrupts daily life.** One of the most common signs of Alzheimer's disease, especially in the early stage, is forgetting recently learned information. Others include forgetting important dates or events, asking for the same information over and over, and increasingly needing to rely on aides (e.g., reminder notes or electronic devices) or family members for things they used to handle on their own.

What's a typical age-related change? Sometimes forgetting names or appointments, but remembering them later.

_____

_____

_____

☐ **2. Challenges in planning or solving problems.** Some people may experience changes in their ability to develop and follow a plan or work with numbers. They may have trouble following a familiar recipe or keeping track of monthly bills. They may have difficulty concentrating and take much longer to do things than they did before.

What's a typical age-related change? Making occasional errors when balancing a checkbook.

_____

_____

_____

☐ **3. Difficulty completing familiar tasks at home, at work, or at leisure.** People with Alzheimer's disease often find it hard to complete daily tasks. Sometimes they may have trouble driving to a familiar location, managing a budget at work, or remembering the rules of a favorite game.

What's a typical age-related change? Occasionally needing help to use the settings on a microwave or to record a television show.

_____

_____

_____

☐ **4. Confusion with time or place.** People with Alzheimer's can lose track of dates, seasons, and the passage of time. They may have trouble understanding something if it is not happening immediately. Sometimes they may forget where they are or how they got there.

What's a typical age-related change? Getting confused about the day of the week but figuring it out later.

_____

_____

_____

☐ **5. Trouble understanding visual images and spatial relationships.** For some people, having vision problems is a sign of Alzheimer's. They may have difficulty reading, judging distance, and determining color or contrast, which may cause problems with driving.

What's a typical age-related change? Vision changes related to cataracts.

_____

_____

_____

☐ **6. New problems with words in speaking or writing.** People with Alzheimer's disease may have trouble following or joining a conversation. They may stop in the middle of a conversation and have no idea how to continue or they may repeat themselves. They may struggle with vocabulary, have problems finding the right word, or call things by the wrong name (e.g., calling a "watch" a "hand clock").

What's a typical age-related change? Sometimes having trouble finding the right word.

_____

_____

_____

☐ **7. Misplacing things and losing the ability to retrace steps.** A person with Alzheimer's may put things in unusual places. They may lose things and be unable to go back over their steps to find them again. Sometimes, they may accuse others of stealing. This may occur more frequently over time.

What's a typical age-related change? Misplacing things from time to time and retracing steps to find them.

_____

_____

_____

☐ **8. Decreased or poor judgment.** People with Alzheimer's may experience changes in judgment or decision making. For example, they may use poor judgment when dealing with money, giving large amounts to telemarketers. They may pay less attention to grooming or keeping themselves clean.
What's a typical age-related change? Making a bad decision once in a while.

_____

_____

_____

☐ **9. Withdrawal from work or social activities.** A person with Alzheimer's disease may start to remove themselves from hobbies, social activities, work projects, or sports. They may have trouble keeping up with a favorite sports team or remembering how to complete a favorite hobby. They may also avoid being social because of the changes they have experienced.
What's a typical age-related change? Sometimes feeling weary of work, family, and social obligations.

_____

_____

_____

☐ **10. Changes in mood and personality.** The mood and personalities of people with Alzheimer's can change. They can become confused, suspicious, depressed, fearful, or anxious. They may be easily upset at home, at work, with friends, or in places where they are out of their comfort zone.
What's a typical age-related change? Developing very specific ways of doing things and becoming irritable when a routine is disrupted.

_____

_____

_____

If you or someone you care about is experiencing any of the ten warning signs of Alzheimer's disease, please see a doctor to find the cause. Early diagnosis gives you a chance to seek treatment and plan for your future.

The Alzheimer's Association can help. Visit http://alz.org/10signs or call 800-272-3900 (TTY: 866-403-3073).

2. Static Declines After a Stroke or Brain Injury

Brain damage from a bump on the head, stroke, or heart attack is not good, but I want to dispel a commonly held false belief about these conditions. Note that I'm going to refer to this category as "injury," but also know that I am using that term inclusively for other injuries from stroke, anoxia (no oxygen to the brain for a while), remitting MS (as opposed to the progressive forms of multiple sclerosis, the remitting types involve just one or a few "flare-ups" that damage nerve tissue but then stop), and so forth.

Far too many people limit themselves after a static injury by believing that they have lit the fuse on a progressive dementia and that their functioning is bound to worsen over time. Plant this firmly in your brain: *The opposite is more likely to be true.* Your first day is usually your worst day. Over time you can expect your cognitive skills to continue getting better. While most recovery happens within the first twelve to twenty-four months, there is now lots of evidence showing that people continue improving five and even ten years after an injury. Rehabilitation isn't passive or easy. These people work hard to regain skills, but through neuroplasticity and active effort, they continue getting better. Therefore, the general course of recovery after an injury is *upward.* Downward is not expected.

I've met a lot of people who experienced one or two mild concussions and worry themselves sick that they are getting that dreaded chronic traumatic encephalopathy (CTE) that so many NFL players are found to have in their brains. The thing is, we still don't know much about CTE, and most of us aren't NFL players. The science on CTE is still in its infancy, at the case study level (Asken et al. 2017). As of the writing of this book, no studies have followed people over time to map the course of CTE, and thus no clinical syndrome can truly be said to have been identified. Please be wary of news reports that claim that certain behaviors, like murder, were "caused by CTE." We simply do not have the science to support these claims. Brain injuries may lower your brain and cognitive reserve (described in the next chapter), increasing your risk for dementia down the line, but lots of other things do this as well. Please don't panic and assume that your concussion has started you down the scary dementia spiral because, as you will see in the next section, your beliefs about your brain matter—a lot.

If you don't correct the underlying problem that caused the injury in the first place though, you could be on the road to something more progressive. Continuing to put your brain at risk for more concussions doesn't help. Having a stroke does increase your risk of having another, especially if the underlying cause—such as high blood pressure, a heart valve issue, or a clotting disorder—isn't treated effectively.

Static or Progressive? Which is it?

Some conditions could go either way. For example, multiple sclerosis (MS) is an autoimmune disorder that damages the white matter (the insulation on your nerve pathways) in your brain and other parts of your nervous system, disrupting the electrical signaling of nerve cells throughout the body, brain, and spinal cord. This matters because these electrical signals are how neurons communicate with one another. There are different types of MS though, so in some cases the damage happens only once or a few times and stops, it remits, or the damage can be progressive. The same is true with epilepsy. Every seizure has the potential to damage some brain cells, but if your seizures are controlled, then the potential for ongoing damage is reduced.

Common Static Injuries and Risk Factors Checklist

Check all that apply to you.

Common static injuries:

- ☐ Stroke
- ☐ TIA (transient ischemic attack), a ministroke with neurological symptoms resolving on their own within twenty-four hours
- ☐ Traumatic brain injury (TBI)
- ☐ Concussion or mild traumatic brain injury (mTBI)
- ☐ Concussion blast injury (being near an explosion)
- ☐ Gunshot wound
- ☐ Heart failure
- ☐ Carbon monoxide poisoning
- ☐ Brain surgery
- ☐ Brain infection from encephalitis or encephalopathy
- ☐ Autoimmune response, such as MS, sarcoidosis, lupus

Risk factors:

- ☐ Seizures
- ☐ Heart disease
- ☐ Peripheral artery disease (PAD, blood clots that typically form in the legs)
- ☐ Atrial fibrillation (AFib)
- ☐ Arteriosclerosis (hardening of the arteries)
- ☐ Diabetes
- ☐ Hypertension

3. Anxiety, Trauma, and False Beliefs

A big benefit of receiving a neuropsychological assessment is having a psychologist determine objectively if your memory is as bad as you think. You may learn from a neuropsychologist that you are working yourself up over nothing, which itself can get in the way of your memory. Neuropsychologists see lots of people who are suffering, worried about their memories, but memory is not the root of the problem. A neuropsychologist can tell you if your memory complaints are the result of anxiety, depression, psychological trauma, insecurity, or even false beliefs. Self-fulfilling prophesies are very real and very powerful. If you believe that your memory sucks, then it tends to fail you.

I see the impact of these false beliefs in my clinic *a lot* because it is one of the cornerstones on which I built my practice. We treat people (referred by other neuropsychologists) to help them develop a better relationship with their emotions and their memories.

We also commonly see people who have experienced relatively mild concussions where it is unlikely that brain cells were permanently damaged, but over time these patients are not recovering as expected. For many, the brain has likely recovered, but the experience of having had a period when their brain didn't work so well causes them to become hypervigilant of any potential sign of long-term damage.

No matter the reason, what I hear most often from people worried about their brains is a hefty dose of self-criticism. People are fearful of appearing dumb, so in turn they worry a lot about their memories. That worry in turn affects memory. It can be challenging to help people understand that it is in fact the worry and associated physical symptoms of anxiety that are causing their memory glitches. People are often defensive about their emotions. Many would rather have something wrong with their brain than admit that they are struggling emotionally or having relationship problems.

The good news is that emotions are making a comeback. We are consistently better understanding their usefulness. Improving your EQ (emotional intelligence) can dramatically improve your memory, and it's becoming cool now to improve your social and emotional intelligence (SEI).

What Are False Beliefs?

False beliefs are beliefs that people have about their memories that are not grounded in facts. They are often fear based, and many come from the media, like the belief that having one or two concussions is a death sentence. Think about your strongly held political or religious beliefs. How open are you to considering the other side? These types of firmly held beliefs are difficult to challenge, but challenging them is essential in a lot of cases, especially when you are using these beliefs to limit your potential.

While it's true that memory declines with age, be careful about viewing the past through rose-colored glasses. Lots of people over forty forget that they also forgot in their twenties. So now when they notice one of the thousands or quite possibly millions of memory errors that our brains make naturally every day, they worry. There was a lot of forgetting back then, but the glitches didn't hold as much meaning as they do now. You did have fewer glitches back then, but your memory was never perfect. We know that from over forty years of research (Loftus 2005). Let's all say it together, *"Memory is not perfect."* Eyewitness testimony is very often trumped by forensic evidence because memory is so imperfect (and I should know; I watch a lot of *Forensic Files*).

Self-Assessment: Worrying About Your Brain

Are you worried about your memory more than other people think you need to be?	Y / N
Are you afraid of being dumb?	Y / N
Do you criticize yourself or your memory?	Y / N
Do you feel physical symptoms of anxiety, like a pit in your stomach or light-headedness, when you can't remember something?	Y / N
Has anyone ever said that you tend to criticize yourself?	Y / N
Do you avoid things that you fear might prove once and for all that you aren't good enough or smart enough?	Y / N
Do you avoid activities that remind you of your memory or thinking concentration challenges, like reading?	Y / N
When you can't come up with the word you want, do you sometimes get flashes of catastrophic ideas or images, like being wheeled into the nursing home?	Y / N

If you answered yes to any of the above, then worry may be a big source of your struggle. I still recommend getting checked out by a neuropsychologist to make sure something bigger isn't happening, but in either case, I want you to pay extra special attention to the emotional components of this book.

Let's Dig Even Deeper

What would it mean to you to know that your memory is not sharp? What might happen if it turned out you weren't as smart as you thought you were? Don't censor yourself; really try to capture any and all thoughts even if they seem a little out there to you or you don't believe them when you say them out loud; they all matter.

Cindy wrote: It would mean that people are going to take advantage of me because I'm not smart enough to take care of myself. I'd be so embarrassed too. My family always really valued being smart; I would feel unworthy.

_____

_____

_____

_____

_____

_____

4. Health Conditions and Lifestyle Patterns That Dull Your Skills

As you probably gathered from the long checklist at the beginning of this chapter, there are a lot of chemical, health, and lifestyle factors that can affect your memory as well. The seven skills in the second half of the book are devoted to helping you modify many of these factors. Therefore, I won't go into a lot of detail now, but suffice it to say that losing sleep, drinking a lot, downing a bunch of Oreos, popping a sleeping pill, being overcommitted and disorganized, not feeling like you matter, and never ever moving your body can have a big impact on your memory.

Let's Check In

I've thrown a lot of new info at you, so I'd like you to jot down some of your feelings so far.

Cindy wrote: I'm a little freaked out and a little pissed off that I didn't know a lot of this stuff before. I'm also feeling excited, but scared because what if I can't do this stuff she's recommending?

Your feelings: _____

_____

_____

_____

_____

Do you feel better or worse knowing that there are different sources of memory loss? What are some of your thoughts on this?

_____

_____

_____

_____

_____

_____

Were the self-assessments helpful? Do you fall into one of the categories? Did this surprise you? For example, does it seem that you have false beliefs, but that feels overwhelming and you don't like it? Or are you even more convinced now that you have a progressive decline, and you are scared out of your mind? Log your thoughts here.

_____

_____

_____

_____

_____

_____

Your First Memory Strategy: Pay Attention

I know the subtitle of this book promises you seven skills to building a better memory, but let's face it, there are many more than seven skills for improving memory. I feel like if I only give you seven, then I will be ripping you off. I want to teach you another memory strategy now that you can practice along the way.

Your first memory strategy is to build up another cognitive skill that is an essential gateway to your memory. *Your memory is only as good as your attention.* You can't hope to remember something you didn't pay attention to in the first place, right? It's really not fair to expect yourself to remember something you never captured because you were off in La La Land. So, the first place to start in building a better memory is to start by building better focus.

Attention is a skill that is vulnerable to a lot of external and internal forces. Attention is affected by distractions, interruptions, boredom, overstimulation, overcomplexity, multitasking, lack of motivation, tiredness—you name it. It's also the first skill that is most influenced by things happening in the body, like chronic fatigue, chronic pain, low oxygen saturation, as well as emotional states like anxiety, depression, and excitement.

What Are Some Things That Block Your Attention?

Cindy wrote: Oh, so maybe the reason I'm having so much trouble is because I stayed up super late last night, or maybe it was that third drink. What if it's my stress level? I do tend to be inside my head a lot.

1. _____

2. _____

3. _____

4. _____

5. _____

6. _____

7. _____

8. _____

9. _____

10. _____

Better Attention Idea Checklist

Below is a list of common recommendations for improving attention. Check the ones that you would like to implement. (*You can also download this exercise as a printable worksheet at http://newharbinger.com/47438.*)

- ☐ Intend to pay attention
- ☐ Prepare to pay attention
- ☐ Conserve energy
- ☐ Eliminate distractions
- ☐ Limit interruptions
- ☐ Get more sleep
- ☐ Get better sleep
- ☐ Clear out mental clutter
- ☐ Meditate
- ☐ Engage in better self-care
- ☐ Move around to build up energy
- ☐ Speed up
- ☐ Slow down
- ☐ "Pay" attention—like money, really invest in this skill; give it an active effort
- ☐ Bribe yourself with rewards for paying attention or staying on task
- ☐ Talk to yourself to stay on task
- ☐ Listen actively
- ☐ Simplify things
- ☐ Take breaks
- ☐ Pace yourself
- ☐ Allow more time
- ☐ Allow less time (set a deadline)
- ☐ Ask for and receive help

Set Your Attention Intention

Now, set your intention for attention. From the list above, pick two of the strategies that you checked and want to work on. Write them in the spaces below.

1. Identify the low-hanging fruit.

Which one on the list seems like a "no-big-deal step"? Pick something that you don't think will be that challenging to implement and may even deliver the biggest return on your investment. Then determine a plan to implement it.

Cindy's no-big-deal step: **Pay attention**

Cindy's plan-to-implement strategy: **I will look at people straight in the eye when they are talking, and not touch my phone.**

Your no-big-deal step: _____

Your plan-to-implement strategy: _____

_____

_____

_____

_____

_____

2. Now challenge yourself a bit.

Pick one strategy that will take more effort. This may require you to be more assertive (asking people to quiet down or give you space), or it may require extra concentration (stopping multitasking or internal chatter).

Cindy's goal: **Make my kids leave the room when I need to focus.**

Cindy's plan-to-implement strategy: **I will sit them down ahead of time and explain why it's important to me.**

Your goal: _____

Your plan-to-implement strategy: _____

_____

_____

_____

_____

_____

Chapter 3

Memory in the Brain

In this chapter, you will learn that different brain systems are responsible for different types of memories. I hope this will help you appreciate the fact that memory is not a singular skill housed in only one part of the brain but rather a few skills spread across the brain. Furthermore, a good memory relies on other cognitive skills, like paying attention and being organized, which rely on even more brain structures. By learning how to respect, nurture, and train a few component brain parts, you will build a better memory.

I've tried to make the brain sections that follow as readable as possible, but you may find some parts to be fairly technical. I've included a lot of details on purpose in keeping with the neuroscience approach. To support you with all of this, I've built in a memory strategy designed to help you distill and then digest the parts most important to you.

WOPR: An Evidence-Based Memory-Encoding Treatment

I want to teach you a technique that, when used as part of a bigger rehabilitation training program, has been shown to be effective in improving memory in people with mild to moderate memory declines (Stringer 2007b). It hails from a program called Ecologically Oriented Neurorehabilitation of Memory (EON-MEM), developed by Anthony Stringer (2007a) a neuropsychologist at Emory University. Mental health and rehabilitation professionals can buy the EON-MEM program workbooks to use with their patients. I'm including a snippet of those skills here. If you are interested in completing the entire twenty-one-week evidence-based program, I encourage you to seek out a provider who can offer you the training.

We will use the four-step method from Dr. Stringer's EON-MEM program to help you form new memories using the acronym WOPR (pronounced "whopper," like the burger or the malted milk balls). WOPR stands for write, organize, picture, and rehearse. After a little training in WOPR, you'll use WOPR throughout this chapter and the next two chapters to help you better remember what you're learning.[1]

---

1   Selected material from the EON-MEM copyright © 2007 by Western Psychological Services. Reprinted by New Harbinger Publications by permission of WPS. Not to be reprinted in whole or in part for any additional purpose without the expressed, written permission of the publisher (rights@wpspublish.com). All rights reserved.

Drilling WOPR

First, I want to make sure you fully absorb the acronym, so I want you to write *WOPR* five times (write the actual acronym to "drill it" for yourself, like doing basketball drills):

_____

_____

_____

_____

_____

Now fill in the blanks:

W = _____   W = _____

O = _____   O = _____

P = _____   P = _____

R = _____   R = _____

W = _____   W = _____

O = _____   O = _____

P = _____   P = _____

R = _____   R = _____

Write

The first step in WOPR is write things down. Often we expect too much of our memories, and we get mad when we don't immediately memorize something. Memory is not perfect, and you can forget a lot of information very rapidly. Writing things down is an essential first step to memory enhancement, and when you are writing, paraphrasing helps. "Paraphrasing" simply means putting information into your own words. You will use paraphrasing as you take notes in these dense neuroscience chapters. If you want to use simple language or off-the-wall analogies, go ahead. Both can be really effective. You're not teaching a neuroscience class at Harvard. You're teaching yourself about the brain, so use language and analogies you understand and that resonate with you.

Why is it important to write things down and paraphrase? (Use your own words.)

_____

_____

_____

_____

Organize

Step 2 of WOPR is to organize. Once you've taken some notes, you will go back and organize the information you've written. If your notes are more narrative and not bullet points or a numbered outline, then take a second pass and make an outline or a bullet list to organize the information. Another great step in organizing is to make associations or to link the information to something you already know. If you make some linkages, no matter how "weird" they might seem to other people, note those linkages for yourself in your outline or bullet list.

- _____

- _____

- _____

Picture (Make Visual Notes)

Step 3 of WOPR is to picture. Seeing information in your mind is a very powerful memory strategy. I explain why in the memory sections below. So make some doodles or diagrams or emojis. Make the information visual or picturesque. You can also take a mental snapshot of the outline or bullets you made in the organize step, and see it inside your mind. Try it. Look at the text or at an image and then close your eyes. Did you "see" it behind your eyelids?

Draw a picture of WOPR to help you visualize the acronym. It can be whatever you want. You can write the letters in a fancy way or draw a picture of a hamburger or a carton of malted milk balls. Get creative.

Rehearse

Don't forget that practice makes perfect, the operative word being "practice." No self-respecting ballerina would be caught dead trying to perform a routine after just seeing it once and never rehearsing it, right? Repeat the information to yourself or to someone else a few times. Drill or quiz yourself on the lists that you've made. Picture those visual images over and over. Do it throughout the day. Depending on your age and level of memory function, you may need to rehearse a bit of information ten to fifteen times or more before it really sticks, so keep rehearsing.

In the next section, you'll use WOPR to help you learn the neuroscience underlying how memory works in the brain. Knowing how memory works will help you better control its function.

Where Is Memory in the Brain?

The question of where memory lives in the brain would be easier to answer if memory were a single thing, but it's not. There are several different types of memory housed in different parts of the brain. Furthermore, memory is not a cognitive skill that can function alone. It relies on other brain skills, like attention and executive function, to operate. But don't fret. My goal is to help unravel this mystery.

Short-Term Memory (aka Attention and Working Memory)

Neuroscientists conceptualize short-term memory quite differently from what most people discuss colloquially. Any memory that you retain for longer than thirty seconds is a long-term memory. You might be thinking, *Huh? Really? So, you're saying that what I remember from the last paragraph is the same as what I learned in kindergarten?* It's true, pretty much.

In neuroscience, short-term memory is more of an attention skill than a memory skill. Just to confuse things, we now call it "working memory." Working memory is the new short-term memory. Working memory is a short-term platform where you hold new information in your mind just long enough to do something with it. If you don't write it down, repeat it, or store it as a long-term memory, then, *swoosh*, it goes away. Working memory is the intersection of attention and memory, which means you have to pay attention to have a good memory. It also has a limited capacity of seven units on average, plus or minus two from person to person, so you can't hold infinite bits of information in your working memory either. This is why you miss stuff.

Updating short-term memory to "working memory" helps expand our understanding of this system, too, because it's actually a lot cooler than just holding info in your attention so it doesn't disappear. Working memory also allows you to manipulate information in your mind (such as when you figure the tip on a bill) and blend it with old memories (like when making associations between new information and the stuff you already know). There are a couple of different systems within working memory, including what's called the "phonological loop" (mentally hearing information inside your head) and the "visuospatial sketchpad" (seeing it in your mind's eye, Baddeley 2010).

Working memory relies on a small, circular area, about the size of a quarter, on the outer surface of the prefrontal cortex (see figure 1). You can imagine this area on each side of your forehead, about an inch above the outer edges of your eyebrows. Cells in this part of your prefrontal cortex become active when you're holding an image or a thought in your mind (Goldman-Rakic 1995).

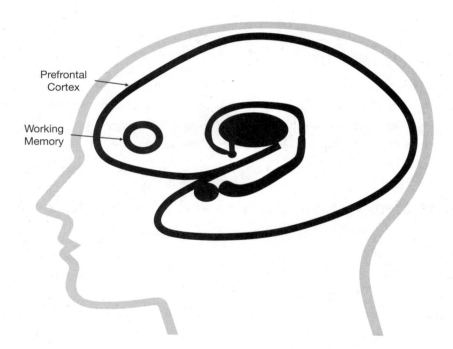

Figure 1. The Working Memory Section of the Prefrontal Cortex

The steps in WOPR really engage the working memory platform. Writing, organizing, picturing, and rehearsing keeps information in your working memory longer, facilitating repeated exposure. "Working" with a new memory inside your working memory (such as manipulating the information through organizing and picturing) gives the long-term storage parts of your brain a better chance to turn it into a long-term memory.

WOPR: Short-Term/Working Memory

Write. What is short-term/working memory? (Paraphrase; put in your own words.)

_____

_____

_____

Quick quiz. How long does short-term memory last? _____ (Add this to your definition if you didn't include it above.)

Organize. Put your definition into a few bullet points.

- _____

- _____

- _____

Picture. Draw a picture of short-term memory. It could be the part of the brain we discussed, or it could be a mental image of very short term. It could take you all of thirty seconds to draw it; be creative.

Rehearse. Practice over and over either your bullet points or your picture, or even picture your bullet points.

Long-Term Memory

Long-term memory is considered either "explicit" or "implicit," and there are basically three types of long-term memory. The first is explicit, and it is the stuff you know you know and you likely remember when you learned it because the learning was an event. Explicit learning is also referred to as "episodic"; like an episode of your favorite TV show, these types of events are things you remember. Explicit learning is also called "declarative" and "semantic" because it involves your memory for facts and information—things you would read in the newspaper, hear from a friend, or learn in school.

The other two types of long-term memory are considered implicit. They develop and operate pretty much outside of your awareness. You may not really know how or when an implicit memory was formed. One type of implicit memory is "procedural memory" or "muscle memory," like habits or riding a bike, and the other type is your "emotional memory."

Three different parts of the brain govern these three different types of memory. Let's dig into each one, but we will be spending a lot more time on the first type since it's the type we think about most when we consider "memory."

Explicit Episodic Memory

There is a network of structures deep inside your brain that allows you to form new, lasting long-term memories for facts and events (explicit episodic memories). These structures work together through a pathway called the Papez circuit, named after the scientist who discovered it (Bhattacharyya 2017). The star of the Papez circuit system is the hippocampus. Most people have two of these, one on each side of the brain, sitting right above your ears. "Hippocampi" is the plural form of the word "hippocampus."

Without the hippocampus, you could still form emotional memories and procedural or muscle memories, but you couldn't form any new explicit episodic memories. We know a lot about the hippocampus from a legendary neurological case of a man named Henry Molaison (Squire 2009). Generations of medical, psychology, and neuroscience students affectionately know him as H. M., as he was identified only by his initials before his death in 2008.

Henry had terrible seizures that his doctors could not control. To stop the seizures, a neurosurgeon removed the hippocampi and some surrounding tissue on both sides of his brain. Brain surgery of this type is still used today, but neurosurgeons now work really hard to not have to remove the hippocampus, especially not both.

From that day forward, Henry could no longer form new explicit memories for facts and events. Every moment was novel. Despite spending decades in relationship with the scientists who studied him, every time he saw them, it was as though they had never met.

Hollywood portrayals of amnesia are almost always wildly inaccurate. The movie character most like H. M. was played by Drew Barrymore in the movie *50 First Dates*, in which her memory reset every night. Unlike her, Henry's memory reset every thirty to ninety seconds, which is what it's like for a person with moderate to severe Alzheimer's disease.

The hippocampal region is attacked early by Alzheimer's disease, so this type of amnesia is a hallmark feature (Imbimbo, Lombard, and Pomara 2005). People call Alzheimer's "short-term memory loss" because memory for recent events is poor, but Alzheimer's is really a *long-term memory* problem. Remember, long-term memory starts at thirty seconds. Alzheimer's *seems* like short-term memory loss because memories from long ago are much stronger than memories from the near term, but they are all long-term memories. The old memories were formed back when the Papez circuit was working. Now it's not working well, and thus new long-term memories are not stored as well as the old ones.

You can have the greatest hippocampi and still have this type of amnesia because you need the entire Papez circuit to be working to encode new memories. Figure 2 shows the Papez circuit, but only the one on the left side of the brain; you have two Papez circuits (and, thus, two of each of the structures shown), one on the right and one on the left.

The hippocampus is connected to the nerve pathway called the fornix, which connects to the mamillary bodies, two very small circular nuclei (collections of cell bodies) right in the middle of your brain that connect to the anterior (or front part of the) thalamus. All four of these structures (hippocampus, fornix, mamillary bodies, and anterior thalamus) must be functional for you to lay down new, explicit long-term memories.

Each structure can be damaged. A stroke or brain tumor could cut or put pressure on the fornix respectively. The mammillary body is sensitive to an extreme thiamine deficiency that can occur in a type of alcoholism called Wernicke-Korsakoff's syndrome. The damage isn't from the alcohol, but because the person drinks so much they forget to eat for many days, depriving the brain of thiamine. The thalamus is an important brain structure. It's like Grand Central Station for your brain in that it is the relay station for many skills, including four out of five senses (not smell), which first travel to the thalamus before going anywhere else in the brain (Fama and Sullivan 2015). Damage to the thalamus, from a tumor or stroke, can disrupt many skills, including the formation of new long-term memories.

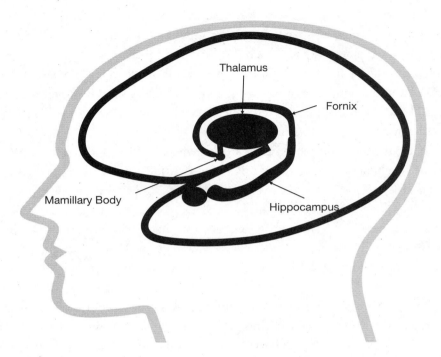

Figure 2. Long-term explicit memory encoding happens in the Papez circuit, which includes the hippocampus, fornix, mamillary body, and thalamus. This figure is meant to be a somewhat three-dimensional representation. The cross section occurs at a bit of a slant, such that structures at the bottom of the figure are farther out toward the edges of your head (the hippocampus is closer to your ear than the middle of your face), whereas structures at the top of the figure are more at the midline (in line with your nose).

WOPR: Long-Term Explicit Memory

Write. What is long-term memory? (Paraphrase; put in your own words.)

_____

_____

Quick quiz. When does long-term memory start? _____ (Add this to your definition if you didn't include it above.)

Organize. Put your definition into a few bullet points.

- _____

- _____

- _____

Picture. Draw a picture of long-term memory. It could be the parts of the brain we discussed, a diagram, or whatever. I bet you can get really creative with the names of the brain structures: Hippocampus—a hippo at college? Mamillary bodies? Fun fact: The word "hippocampus" is Latin for "seahorse."

You can also go to figure 2 and trace the Papez circuit with your finger or a pencil, following the pathway from the hippocampus, up through the fornix to the mamillary bodies, and up into the thalamus. I found that diagramming the pathway or tracing its route through the brain on the figure really helped me memorize the circuit.

Rehearse. Practice your bullet points or your picture, or even picture your bullet points.

Verbal vs. Visual Memory

Did you know that you have two sides to your brain? You're probably thinking, *Yeah, duh. I knew that.* I mention it this way because we often refer to brain structures in the singular, like "the hippocampus," but in reality you have two hippocampi, one on each side of your brain. Almost every brain structure is duplicated; one on the left, one on the right. You have two complete Papez circuits, which is important to remember because each side handles the long-term storage of two different types of information.

For most people, even most left-handed people, language lives in the left hemisphere of the brain (Corballis 2014). There is some variation, but not as much as you might think. Since language is on the left, only the left Papez circuit forms new memories for auditory, verbal, and language-based information. Your right Papez circuit is responsible for learning *visual* information. This is the home of your "mind's eye" and your "cognitive map" (being able to give directions to someone from memory).

Because humans have evolved to read, write, and speak, we tend to overtax our left-hemisphere memory circuit. We tell ourselves to remember things verbally, with lots of internal, verbal chatter. One very effective way to boost your memory is to call upon your right-hemisphere memory circuit to remember things visually, using the picture step of WOPR. Many people don't think to use this right circuit, but visualization strategies are remarkably effective. Some argue that they may even be more effective than verbal memories because we've probably had visual memory longer. Remember cavemen? It doesn't seem likely that they spoke to each other, but they knew where all the berries were.

The hemispheres are specialized for other types of information as well, not just language versus visual, which may be why language ended up in the left hemisphere. The left hemisphere is partial to details and processes information logically and in a linear way, focusing on the past, the future, and ourselves. The right hemisphere is partial to information that is more about the big picture, the whole, and the world outside of ourselves. So, remember, left is for language, linear, and logic, and right is for visual, big picture, and the world.

WOPR: Visual vs. Verbal Encoding

Write and organize. For most people, which type of memory is encoded on which side of the brain, and what types of information do the hemispheres favor?

Left	Right

Picture. Spend a moment visualizing memories getting encoded in the brain through the Papez circuit, such as words getting stored on the left side and images getting stored on the right side. Draw pictures for the types of memories that each hemisphere encodes.

Left	Right

Rehearse. Practice over and over your pictures and lists.

Recall of Long-Term Explicit Memories

You can have the best Papez circuit in the world and still have memory problems. This is because the hippocampus and other structures within the Papez circuit are only responsible for helping you *put new memories into your brain*, or what we call "encoding." Pulling memories out of your brain, involves an entirely different skill called "recall," which relies on a different part of your brain.

Recall depends on your prefrontal cortex, the outer covering of the brain at the front (see figure 3), which is responsible for executive functions, skills like planning, organizing, and inhibiting (Cummings 1993). Executive skills help you encode memories because they help organize information to store it better, like the organize step in WOPR. The frontal lobes are also responsible for "going and getting" the memory later, or *recall*. It's not just the prefrontal cortex that is needed for memory recall. The cortex is where the cell bodies of the neurons live, and recall relies on the "axons" (the long arms or nerve fibers of the neuron, also known as "white matter pathways") that connect the frontal lobes to other parts of the brain. I call these the "go get it" pathways because they go fetch the memory for recall.

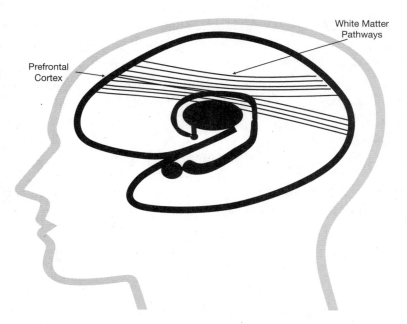

Figure 3. Recall of explicit memories relies on the broader prefrontal cortex (PFC) and the white matter (axonal or nerve) pathways ("go get it" pathways) connecting the PFC with other parts of the brain.

Recall Strategies

Ever hear of a "senior moment"? This is that tip-of-the-tongue phenomenon when people can't come up with the name of that restaurant they ate at last week. The memory is usually in their brain; they are just struggling to recall it. I often hear people beat themselves up over this, but I want you to stop doing that because it doesn't help.

When you are trying to remember that new thing you learned, I want you to use these strategies adapted from the cognitive rehabilitation program CogSMART (Twamley et al. 2012, 66).

1. Relax.

   A lot of people panic when they have a "senior moment," but that's probably the worst thing you can do. Anxiety interferes with your ability to retrieve information. Work to calm your body and mind when your recall is stuck. This will increase your chances of accessing the information. Thinking harder won't.

2. Retrace your steps.

   To retrieve a lost item or access a detail about a past event, mentally retrace your steps and think about the events leading up to when you last had the item.

3. Search the alphabet.

   To remember a word or a name, go through the alphabet, starting with *A*, and ask yourself, "Does it start with *A*? Does it start with *B*?" and so on.

4. Recreate the context.

   As Twamley and colleagues (2012) suggest, "This is a good strategy when you can't remember where you were or what you were doing when you learned the information. For example, if you remember that you were eating at a certain restaurant when your friend told you about a class that you wanted to take, recreate that context. Either imagine the restaurant or actually go there, and it will be easier for you to remember the details about the class" (66).

5. Stick to a structured schedule.

   Identify your daily routine and schedule things you want to do but often have difficulty remembering to do or motivating yourself to do (such as medications, exercise, and so forth).

WOPR: Recall

Write. What is recall? (Paraphrase; put in your own words.)

_____

_____

List some steps that you plan to take the next time your recall gets "stuck" and you can't access what you want to remember.

_____

_____

_____

_____

Organize. Put your definition into a few bullet points.

- _____

- _____

- _____

Picture. Draw a picture of recall. It could be the parts of the brain we discussed, a diagram, the "go get it" pathways, and so on.

Rehearse. Practice over and over either your bullet points or your picture, or even picture your bullet points.

Implicit Procedural (Muscle) Memory

Implicit memories are memories you may not remember "creating." You may not even understand why they exist, like certain habits or associations, such as when you feel faint opening your bank balance. The first type of implicit memory is procedural, or muscle, memory. These memories are made up of habits or automatic skills that you "just do" and don't really think about, like riding a bike. They live in the middle of your brain in a circuit of structures called the basal ganglia (Wise 1996). The basal ganglia might sound like a yummy Thai dish, but it's a complicated collection of "nuclei" (groups of cell bodies) that, in concert with the thalamus, help you perform habits, routines, and coordinated muscle movements.

Diseases that are associated with a disruption in the function of the basal ganglia include Parkinson's disease (PD) and obsessive-compulsive disorder (OCD) (Harbishettar et al. 2005). In PD the motor programs lose their coordination, leading to tremors, balance problems, and freezing in place. In OCD the basal ganglia is overactive, leading to rigid routines that are difficult to break.

In Alzheimer's disease, the basal ganglia is spared relatively early on (Vitanova et al. 2019), so an effective way to intervene in rehabilitation is to work to establish new habits and routines that can compensate for the changes in episodic memory.

The basal ganglia is not trained "didactically" (like hearing a lecture), so reading about a new memory technique will not lead to changes in your basal ganglia. You must train it through practice and repetition; think habits and routines.

WOPR: Procedural Memories

Write. What is procedural memory? (Paraphrase; put in your own words.)

_____

_____

Organize. Put your definition into a few bullet points.

- _____

- _____

- _____

Picture. Draw pictures of different types of procedural memories, like biking or running. You could look up images of the basal ganglia online and draw out the network. You could draw that basal ganglia Thai dish that we are all dreaming about—whatever will help you remember details about this type of implicit memory.

Rehearse. Practice over and over either your bullet points or your pictures, or even picture your bullet points.

Implicit Emotional Memory

The third type of long-term memory, also implicit, is emotional memory. These memories form in the amygdala (plural: "amygdalae"), two very small, almond shaped structures that sit right in front of each hippocampus, right above your ears. The amygdalae are your fear detectors. They are constantly monitoring your environment, which includes your internal thoughts, and when one of them decides something is scary, they trigger important brain and body systems to kick into high gear very quickly to help you respond, automatically.

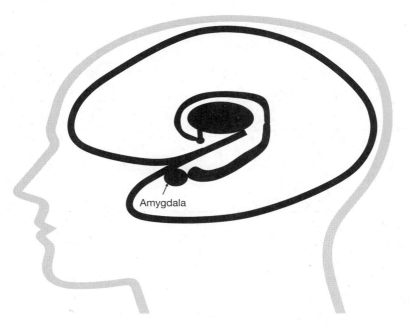

Figure 4. The amygdala is responsible for creating and storing emotional
memories through associations that are housed inside the amygdala.

We will talk more about the stress response later. What I want you to know now is that the amygdala stores your emotional memories. It makes associations between what it thinks will kill you and things that really can kill you and acts accordingly. You can retrain your amygdala, which is exciting, but like your basal ganglia, it doesn't learn through webinars or book reading; it learns through conditioning, associations, or parings. The amygdala doesn't speak English. Training it takes a whole different approach (specifically through exposure to that which is scary).

WOPR: Emotional Memory

Write. What is emotional memory? (Paraphrase; put in your own words.)

_____

_____

Quick quiz. Where do emotional memories live in the brain? _____

Organize. Put your definition into a few bullet points.

- _____

- _____

- _____

Picture. Draw a picture related to emotional memory or the amygdala. (Fun fact: "Amygdala" is Latin for "almond.")

[ ]

Rehearse. Practice over and over either your bullet points or your picture, or even picture your bullet points.

Now that you know that there are multiple types of memories and memory systems, each handling different types of information, you are now better equipped to start working with your brain to improve your memory. Depending on what's going on with your brain, whether it be normal life, aging, a history of trauma, brain injury, or Alzheimer's disease, you can customize your approach to your specific memory challenges to help you improve your memory performance.

Chapter 4

Cognitive Reserve: A Household Name

Two important scientific theories have turned the field of neuroscience upside down, providing a whole new level of hope for improving memory. These are bona fide scientific theories, born out of the scientific method. They summarize the results of scientific data across a range of studies.

In this chapter, I will share with you the background about cognitive reserve, the first theory, and the things that are known to deplete it. Throughout the rest of the book, you will learn how to beef up your cognitive reserve by leveraging positive brain plasticity (the second important neuroscience theory, which is described in the next chapter). Cognitive reserve describes the physical manifestations—the "what"—you need for a strong memory throughout your life, and brain plasticity (also called neuroplasticity) describes "how" you get it, so let's dig in.

A Story About Brains

The best way I've found to introduce cognitive reserve is to start by telling a story about brains. In the late 1980s, a group of researchers asked adults in their eighties to donate their brains when they died (Katzman et al. 1989). The researchers knew which participants had memory problems at the end of their lives and which did not, and they had a fair amount of information about how the participants had lived their lives. Some of the people were sharp as a tack when they died, while others had very advanced memory loss, struggling to care for themselves or remember loved ones. The researchers wanted to know if they could tell which brains belonged to which group by measuring the amount of Alzheimer's disease growing in the brains of a subsample of the participants. They did a blind count of the beta-amyloid plaques, one of the two hallmark features of Alzheimer's disease pathology. (The other pathology is called neurofibrillary tau tangles, but those were not counted in this study.) What do you think they found? Venture a guess.

Do you think the people with advanced dementia had _____ than the people who were sharp as a tack?

   a.   more plaque

   b.   less plaque

   c.   the same amount of plaque

The answer is c, the same amount of plaque. If you guessed more plaque, you're not alone. Many people assume this, but the researchers found significant amounts of Alzheimer's disease plaque in the brains of sharp people, the same as those with advanced dementia.

The researchers (perhaps like yourself) were rather puzzled, so they sought to see if there *was* something different about the brains of the people who were sharp as a tack that might explain this, and they found a difference. The people who were sharper when they died had bigger brains. Brain size is measured a few different ways across different studies, but it includes mass (weight), volume (size), and cell counts (how many neurons per square millimeter). The sharp people had more brain left over, which seemed to allow them to ward off the visible signs of memory decline, despite all the Alzheimer's growing in their brains. It also turned out that the sharp people had been more active throughout their lives, not just intellectually (by reading more, advancing farther in their careers, and so forth) but also physically and socially. The way these sharp people had lived their lives really seemed to make a bigger difference in their risk for memory loss than the amount of Alzheimer's plaque growing in their brains.

Throughout the 1990s similar data was also emerging from other types of brain damage, such as stroke and traumatic brain injury. We still can't predict how much skill loss a person will experience based on the size of a stroke or the severity of a brain injury. Some people experience small strokes and lose lots of skills, while others with big strokes make remarkable recoveries. There are a lot of factors that go into this, but one big factor is how much brain the person has to lose in the first place.

The Birth of a New Theory

Noticing this evidence, a neuropsychologist at Columbia University named Yakov Stern (2002) published a series of papers starting in the year 2000 summarizing this evidence and proposing the theory of cognitive reserve. This theory synthesized and explained what scientists were seeing across diseases and injuries. It explains that people differ in the number of cells and skills they have stored in their brain banks, and this, *more than disease or injury* in many cases, predicts how early a person will encounter a memory problem. Put another way, *the more cells and skills you have stored in your brain bank, the more you have to lose before crossing over the "dementia threshold"* (represented by the horizontal line on figure 5), which is the point where your memory loss is so bad that we diagnose it as dementia. Having a robust cognitive reserve allows you to better withstand the things that would ravage your memory, allowing you to maintain your memory and independence longer.

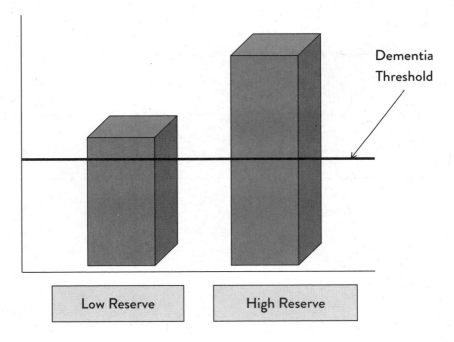

Figure 5. Cognitive Reserve Theory (Stern 2002). The person on the left has a lower cognitive reserve and thus is at greater risk of showing dementia sooner than the person on the right. The person on the right has more brain cells and skills to lose—higher cognitive reserve—before showing signs of dementia.

WOPR: Cognitive Reserve

Write. What is cognitive reserve? (Paraphrase; put in your own words.)

_____

_____

Organize. Put your definition into a few bullet points.

- _____

- _____

- _____

Picture. Draw a picture about cognitive reserve.

Rehearse. Practice over and over either your bullet points or your picture, or even picture your bullet points.

Brain 401(k)

I call cognitive reserve your brain's 401(k) account because it is quite literally your brain's retirement account. I've also made it my professional mission to make "cognitive reserve" a household word, something you think about pretty much every day as you make countless choices. I want you to think about it in much the same way you think about your blood pressure, your weight, your cholesterol levels, and so forth. Why? Because *you can control it!*

Scientific disclaimer: Well, you can control a decent amount of your cognitive reserve. There do seem to be people who are born with brain trust funds, people with genetically bigger brains. Also, unfortunately you can't go back and relive your twenties and drink less beer. But just like your retirement savings, you can control a decent amount of it, even if you're getting a late start on brain 401(k) investing.

Brain 401(k) "Investing"

Early in the days of understanding cognitive reserve, the field of neuroscience was still operating under a very different zeitgeist than it is today. Up until the beginning of this century, the zeitgeist about the adult brain was that it was fixed and hardwired. Therefore, the accepted approach to brain health when we first started to understand cognitive reserve was simply to work hard to help people minimize their brain 401(k) losses. The best advice we had in the early 2000s were things like "Don't bump your head."

However, we have since learned that you can also actively invest in your brain 401(k) throughout your entire life. You can *make contributions to your brain's retirement account* and build yourself a bigger brain that is more resistant to memory loss. I want people across the entire life span thinking about cognitive reserve, because you are either investing in or deducting from your brain 401(k) throughout your entire life.

Brain 401(k) Investing Pays Dividends

The remainder of this book is peppered with solutions to help you maximize your brain 401(k) investing, but you're probably thinking, *I care what happens to my brain when I'm eighty, but I bought this book because I need memory help now.* Well you're in luck! Like any good financial investment strategy, brain 401(k) investing not only helps you build a solid brain portfolio down the line, but these investment strategies also *pay dividends.* Each of the strategies presented in this book are known to have long-term benefits for brain health, and most also provide short-term benefits in helping you have a sharper memory *now.*

Assessing Your Brain 401(k) Portfolio

Let's get a sense of your baseline brain 401(k) investing portfolio. Rate yourself on a scale from 0 to 100 for how well you think you are doing right now in each of the lifestyle areas listed on the bar graph below. Then shade in each bar to reflect that percentage. For example, *I'm giving about 90 percent effort to social support, but only about 30 percent to physical activity.*

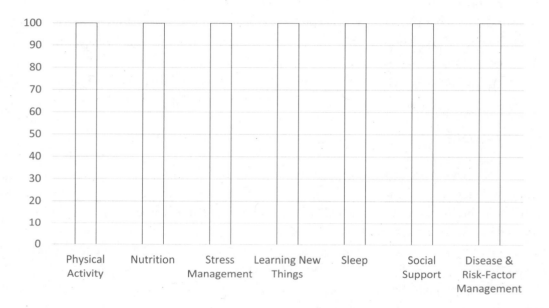

Figure 6. Your Brain 401(k) Portfolio

Minimizing Losses: Some Ugly Truths

Before digging into ways to maximize your investments, it's important that we detour for a bit to talk about some things that can deplete your brain 401(k). I often get so excited about the possibilities of brain 401(k) investing that I gloss right over bad brain investments. You might think of the following list as toxic assets, maybe like a high-interest credit card balance.

The *Lancet Commissions*, a top science journal that "commissions" large-scale reviews, released a thorough analysis of the biggest "potentially modifiable risk factors" for dementia (Livingston et al. 2017). These are health and lifestyle patterns that increase your risk for dementia by eating away at your brain 401(k). Be on the lookout for the following ten things that are known to deplete your brain 401(k) and thus increase your risk for memory loss down the line. This section ends with a self-assessment, so you can get a better sense of your own risk level.

1. Hearing Loss

It is especially detrimental if you lose your hearing in the middle of your life, your forties or fifties, for example, and don't do something about it, but hearing loss can be a risk factor for dementia at any age (Livingston et al. 2017). Hearing loss, and the associated social isolation that often follows, deprives your brain of much-needed stimulation. When there is less input coming into your brain from your ears, your brain cells have less to respond to, potentially leading to atrophy through "use it or lose it." Correcting hearing loss often opens the world back up to people and provides a much wider bandwidth of signal to the brain. Cross your fingers that this new evidence will finally compel American insurance companies to cover hearing aids. If you've been putting off getting your hearing tested or you forget to wear your hearing aids, knowing this link may boost your motivation. In either case, you also don't have to become a wallflower just because you're struggling to hear. There are lots of ways to connect with people and stay active.

2. Obesity

Thank goodness many cultures are combating fat phobia, which is the discriminatory attitude about size that leads to intense fear or shame about being fat and discriminatory policies, like having to purchase an extra seat on an airplane. Trying to control obesity through shame is *not* helpful, and thin does not always equal healthy. At the same time, we can't ignore the evidence that obesity, particularly in the middle part of a person's life, is a known risk factor for dementia (Livingston et al. 2017).

The impact of obesity on the brain is largely indirect and potentially modifiable. It's really less about size and more about health. The ways in which we become and stay obese are hard on the brain, such as sitting on the couch eating sugary and fatty foods, not to mention a few cocktails each night. Excess weight increases the risk for brain-damaging conditions, like high blood pressure, sleep apnea, heart disease, and diabetes. Weight isn't the only cause of these conditions. Genetics do tend to play a big role, but we also know that obesity can exacerbate these conditions.

3. Uncontrolled High Blood Pressure

Uncontrolled high blood pressure, or hypertension, can be hard on your brain and memory. The vascular system in your body includes arteries (carrying oxygenated blood from your heart), veins (carrying "used" blood back to your heart), and capillaries (the small vessels at the tips of the system that feed hard-to-reach nooks and crannies). This is a closed system, and too much pressure inside this closed system can damage both the blood vessels themselves and in some cases your brain cells. Damage to the arterial walls can lead to a buildup of plaque in the arteries, and if some of that plaque were to dislodge and block an artery, it can deprive the brain of critical blood flow. Nerve cells do not store their own energy, so any interruption in blood flow to the brain for even a few minutes can cause massive cell death. The intense pressure on the blood vessels in hypertension can also cause brain bleeds. Brain bleeds and blocking the supply of blood flow to the brain are the two types of stroke, and you can have stroke activity without ever knowing it. The middle part of your brain is especially vulnerable to these ministrokes because they are fed by tiny capillaries, which are particularly vulnerable to blockages and bleeds given their small size. Many people with uncontrolled hypertension (and diabetes, see below) go on to develop memory recall problems resulting in what we have traditionally called vascular dementia, now called vascular neurocognitive disorder (American Psychiatric Association 2013).

Regular annual doctors' visits will likely identify high blood pressure, but frequent headaches, light-headedness, dizziness, or tightness in your neck or chest may indicate blood pressure spikes. To get your blood pressure under control, it's best to work with your doctor to address the underlying causes (smoking, obesity, and so forth) for the long term. However, if your doctor prescribes medication, I recommend you use it. Controlling blood pressure is far too critical for your brain health to gamble by not taking it. Lifestyle changes may or may not be successful or may take a long time, resulting in undue damage to your brain. With certain lifestyle changes and health improvements, you could come off the medication later.

4. Smoking

Fortunately, smoking is getting less and less cool, but in a lot of settings it is still very much accepted. It's no secret that smoking is hard on your body. In terms of your brain, smoking deprives your brain of much-needed oxygen and increases your risk for the vascular brain damage we just discussed. Vaping, consuming nicotine via water vapor instead of cigarettes, was initially thought to be safer given that the water vapor likely doesn't deprive your brain of oxygen in the same way smoking does. However, vaping also appears risky given reports of lung damage and unregulated chemical formulas used in vaping products.

I know it can be hard to quit, and I'm not here to shame you. I am here to encourage you. Quitting is possible and much more achievable with professional help. Smoking-cessation clinics have been around for decades, and services seem to be expanding into primary care settings.

Also, don't let your age deter you from quitting. Don't think, *It's too late for me, so what's the point?* because data shows that quitting smoking later in life, even in your seventies, can still dramatically reduce your risk of dementia (Livingston et al. 2017).

5. Depression

Depression robs you of concentration and memory now and in the long run. It can make you feel foggy and unmotivated, plus it's a major risk factor for dementia (Livingston et al. 2017). The stress hormone cortisol is toxic to brain cells, and when you are depressed, this stuff is pumping constantly throughout your body and brain (Andrade and Kumar Rao 2010). Depression is quite treatable though through psychotherapy, meditation, and medication.

It can be well worth the effort to find a really good therapist. You can even do therapy over the phone. If you suffer from depression, I recommend you seek help beyond this book from a licensed mental health professional, particularly if you feel worthless or suicidal. A therapist can help you learn new ways of thinking and ways of being that are known to combat depression.

6. Physical Inactivity

It's going to come up a lot in this book because moving your body may be the best thing you can do for your brain and memory. You're going to think I'm some sort of exercise freak, but I'm not. I struggle with this as much as the next guy. I love the way I feel when I'm more physically active. I'm sharper and more energetic. I also love sleeping in and sitting on the couch watching Netflix. There can be room for both in this life. My goal is to help you develop and stick to a pattern of physical activity that boosts your brain and memory, because being sedentary is a known dementia risk. Yikes!

7. Social Isolation

Social isolation, particularly loneliness, is a major health risk, as bad as smoking by some estimates (Pantell et al. 2013). It is also a known risk factor for dementia, particularly among older adults (Livingston et al. 2017). The theory is that it damages the brain by depriving it of much-needed stimulation; plus, it's a stressor. Modern humans are still social primates. We depend immensely on each other for our survival and comfort. Without adequate social support, you may be seriously limiting your memory potential both now and in the future.

8. Diabetes

Uncontrolled diabetes is hard on your brain because when your blood sugar gets too high, your red blood cells swell up and block the blood flowing down into the tiny capillaries (the small blood vessels at the ends of the arteries) that feed the middle part of your brain. As we saw with high blood pressure above, depriving brain cells (including nerves) of blood flow, even for a couple of minutes, produces massive cell death.

Have you heard of "diabetic neuropathy"? This is the condition wherein a person with diabetes loses feeling or has pain in their fingers and toes, or when a person with diabetes gets kidney (nephropathy) or eye damage (retinopathy)? Well the same thing happens in your brain. What all these parts of the body (fingers, toes, eyes, kidneys, and deep inside the middle brain) have in common is that they are all fed by capillaries. When the red blood cells swell up from the blood sugar spike, they block blood flow to these regions, damaging the nerves. So, if a doctor has told you that the numbness or tingling you feel in your fingers or toes is from neuropathy, you can bet that the same type of damage may be happening in your brain. Diabetes and high blood pressure affect the same part of the brain and affect your memory and recall over time.

In the short term, diabetes also affects your concentration during times of both high blood sugar and low blood sugar. You don't even have to have diabetes to experience this. For many people (me), eating a big slice of cake can cause a buzz that feels similar to that brought on by a glass of wine. When a healthy insulin response kicks in to combat that sugar, you may feel ready for a nap. All of this lowers your concentration and therefore your memory. You don't have to cut out all sugar, but do try to work for some balance.

9. Dropping Out of School

The relationship between the mental stimulation that comes from education and greater cognitive reserve has been clear from the beginning (Katzman et al. 1989). In those early studies of cognitive reserve that Dr. Stern (2002) reviewed, people who led more mentally active lives had higher reserve. Subsequent large-scale reviews suggest that most of the risk comes from a lack of secondary education (no high school) or less. Relative to other factors on this list, this is rather profound (Livingston et al. 2017). There is more to be learned about the relationship between education and brain health, and as you will learn throughout this book, it's never too late to grow your brain. So, if you didn't finish middle school or high school or college or whatever, it's fantastic that you're reading this book! You're taking decisive action now to invest in your brain 401(k) to make up for the past. If, on the other hand, you have a solid educational background, good for you! Keep up the learning, because we have yet to see a point of diminishing returns.

10. Brain Injury

Brain injury can come in many forms: a blow to the head causing a concussion or more serious injury, a stroke, certain medications, seizures, and so forth. I don't wish to contribute to the collective panic regarding concussions. One concussion does not a dementia cocktail make. However, any type of brain trauma can eat away at your cognitive reserve. It can deplete your fund of cells and move your brain 401(k) portfolio closer to that dementia threshold, meaning that if you were to have a stroke later or had Alzheimer's growing in your brain, your resistance might be lower. That seems pretty depressing, so let me also say that by reading this book and doing the exercises, you can work to offset any potential losses in your brain 401(k) to potentially move your portfolio further away from the threshold.

Also, keep in mind that I added brain injury to the list. It did not pan out as a major risk factor in the *Lancet Commissions* review (Livingston et al. 2017), which means that statistically, the other items on this list are a much greater concern for most people. That said, do wear a helmet when you ride a bike or one of the many new motorized scooters and skateboard things, okay?

Brain 401(k) Portfolio Self-Assessment

Earlier in the chapter you estimated your brain 401(k) portfolio, but let's take a moment to assess how you are investing or deducting from your brain 401(k). This self-assessment has not been scientifically validated, and it is important to keep in mind that professionals can't actually quantify anyone's cognitive reserve at this point. This is an exercise in self-awareness, aimed at helping you set the goals that you will work toward throughout the rest of the book.

1. I engage in physical activity (walking, jogging, dancing, and so forth):
   a. daily or almost daily
   b. 3–4 times per week
   c. 1–2 times per week
   d. about once a week
   e. about once a month
   f. never

2. I smoke:
   a. No
   b. Yes

3. I have diabetes that I manage:
   a. I don't have diabetes.
   b. very well
   c. pretty well
   d. not so well
   e. poorly

4. My job or life causes me to learn new things:
   a. daily
   b. weekly
   c. monthly
   d. quarterly
   e. never

5. My stress levels is:

    a.   totally managed because I meditate every day.

    b.   not so bad; I meditate a few times a week.

    c.   okay; I try to relax.

    d.   not bad; I chill with my friends over cocktails.

    e.   high, oh so high; what does it feel like to relax?

6. Hypertension:

    a.   I have never had a high blood pressure reading in my life.

    b.   I have not been diagnosed with high blood pressure.

    c.   I take my blood pressure medication daily and keep a good eye on my numbers.

    d.   I take my blood pressure medication daily but don't really know how well it's working.

    e.   I think my doctor did mention that once or twice, but I don't really stick to taking my medication.

7. My experience with depression is:

    a.   I'm never depressed.

    b.   I've had some trouble, but I'm working on it; I haven't felt blue in a while.

    c.   I get depressed about once a year.

    d.   I'm always depressed.

8. In my spare time, my hobbies are mostly:

    a.   reading, puzzles, intellectual challenges

    b.   watching TV

    c.   playing Candy Crush

    d.   drinking at the bar

9. My social support network is:

    a.   supportive

    b.   drinking buddies

    c.   stressful

    d.   nonexistent—I'm lonely

10. My sleep is:

    a. great! My head hits the pillow each night, and I rock out a solid eight straight, uninterrupted hours.

    b. okay. I typically sleep seven to eight hours, with maybe a couple of interruptions once or twice a week.

    c. meh. I'm usually up for about an hour or two each night.

    d. not great. I really struggle with sleep.

    e. I sleep fine when I take my Xanax (or something similar, including Benadryl).

11. My body mass (weight relative to height; BMI) is in the:

    a. healthy weight range

    b. overweight range

    c. obese range (BMI 30–35)

    d. morbidly obese range (BMI 35+)

12. My diet is:

    a. rich in fish and veggies that are low glycemic, and low in saturated fats

    b. primarily full of veggies and lean protein with the occasional indulgence

    c. primarily fully of veggies and lean protein with near daily indulgences

    d. mostly meat and potatoes

    e. the four food groups: chips, cookies, candy, and soda

13. People complain about my hearing:

    a. never

    b. sometimes

    c. always

    d. I'm not sure; I can't hear them.

14. I've experienced:

    a. no concussions

    b. one mild concussion where I either didn't lose consciousness or only momentarily

    c. one moderate to severe brain injury where I lost consciousness for several minutes or was very disoriented and still cannot recall some events before and after the head injury

    d. a moderate to severe brain injury more than once

    e. more concussions than I can count

15. My level of education is:

    a. doctoral degree

    b. master's degree

    c. bachelor's (four-year) degree

    d. some college but no degree

    e. high school diploma

    f. more than eighth grade but didn't finish high school

    g. less than eighth grade

Here is how scoring for this assessment works: each answer has a point value: a = 1, b = 2, c = 3, and so on. Once each item has a score, add them all together for a total score.

Scoring Results

15–30 points: You're doing great. You're probably already loving this book because it supports and confirms a lot of what you're doing right already. I think you will also enjoy learning more about the details of what you're doing right, and like most high achievers, you are probably also on the lookout for ways to continue improving. Keep up the good work!

31–50 points: You've got some work to do. For the most part, you're hitting the right strides, but your total indicates that you have some risk factors lurking in the corners. Good job being honest. Continue the truth-telling as you work through the book.

51–70 points: I'm so glad you're here. If you do half of the exercises in this book, then you will have made a difference. Your dementia risk is not looking so good. Some of a person's risk comes from family history, but a lot comes from lifestyle, and I think it's fair to say that your lifestyle puts you at a pretty high risk. But you can change! Be kind to yourself. Consider getting some help from your doctor or another professional. Do the work. You can do it!

Just so you know, Cindy scored a 48. She has some work to do.

Jot down some initial plans for addressing your toxic assets and improving your brain 401(k) investing.

Cindy's plan: I don't think I'm losing my hearing, but my kids are complaining a bit. Maybe I'll ask my doctor about this. Thank god I finished high school. But when was the last time I learned something new? I'll look into signing up for a gardening class. Hmm...I wonder if my dizziness is from my blood pressure. It did come out a little high the last couple of times. I'll ask my doctor about that too. I seem to crash in the evening after I eat chocolate-covered pretzels. I will quit buying them and substitute that snack with fruit or nuts.

Your plan: _____

_____

_____

_____

_____

_____

Great job making it through all of this tough stuff. It can be hard to face these harsh realities. Now let's transition into some more of the positive ways you can actively invest in your brain 401(k).

Chapter 5

Build a More Resilient Brain
Through Neuroplasticity

We just reviewed cognitive reserve and the things that deplete it. In this chapter we will focus on building your cognitive reserve through neuroplasticity. Neuroplasticity is the "how" behind the "what" of cognitive reserve, or brain 401(k) investing.

When cognitive reserve theory was first emerging, most neuroscientists still thought that the adult brain was fixed and hardwired. Therefore, a lot of the early focus was placed on minimizing brain 401(k) losses. Mothers would say, "Don't bump your head; those are all the brain cells you're ever going to have," or "Don't drink too much beer; you'll need those brain cells later on."

By and large these recommendations still hold true. Do work to keep your brain cells because they do not regenerate the way skin and bone cells do. But now minimizing losses is only half the story. We now know that *you can actively invest in your brain 401(k) throughout your entire life span* by growing some new brain cells and helping the ones you've had your whole life build more connections and flourish.

Most people who hear that say something like, "What? Are you kidding me? How do I do that? Don't we have all the brains we are ever going to have at twenty, and it's all downhill from there? That's what I was taught in school. This lady has completely fallen off her rocker, which is sad because she really doesn't seem that old. And somebody paid her to write a memory book?" Cue the eye roll.

All kidding aside, this *is* the science most of us were raised on, and it's how we thought about the adult brain for decades. We aren't really sure why we believed this. Perhaps it was because we thought of the brain like a computer, hardwired, and since computers couldn't adapt or rewire themselves, the brain must function this way too.

Well, that way of thinking has been turned on its head (pun intended). Over the last couple of decades, new evidence has emerged that now proves that the adult brain continues to grow and change in positive ways throughout the entire life span. The theory we are talking about here is what we call "positive brain plasticity." Simply defined, "brain plasticity" refers to our new understanding that the adult brain is much more plastic or malleable than we thought. In this chapter, I share what we've learned about the adult brain over the past couple of decades that supports this theory.

Positive Brain Plasticity Facts and Data

As you will see, I believe it's important that you know about this data because it's the foundation on which the neuroscience approach to improving memory is built. I draw upon this science in helping you remold your brain into an impressive memory machine.

1. Adults Grow New Brain Cells

Adults grow new brain cells. Did you know that? Because before 1998, there was zero evidence that the adult brain grew new brain cells (Eriksson et al. 1998), so in science terms, this is pretty new information. Growing new brain cells is called "neurogenesis."

Why were we in the dark about this fact about brain cells for so long? Well, one reason is because you don't grow a lot of them, and they only grow in one small region of the brain, which is in and around the hippocampus. This means they are not growing all over your brain. If you lose the brain cells that control your left leg for instance, you will *not* grow new brain cells there.

There is more to learn about the function of these new baby brain cells, but the fact that they only grow in and around the hippocampus suggests that they play an important role in forming new memories, a fact that you are capitalizing on as you work through this book. Many of the strategies in this book are aimed at helping you grow more of these new brain cells, because you can affect that rate too. You can also affect how long they stick around and how much they help you out.

The discovery of these adult brain cells involves an interesting story about people who survived cancer through radiation treatment and then donated their brain tissue after they died (Eriksson et al. 1998).

Growing new brain cells has nothing to do with cancer or radiation treatment. The radiation treatment simply allowed scientists the opportunity to find these new baby brain cells. This is because when your body goes through radiation treatment, some of the genetic information in your cells (the RNA) becomes "morphed" or recoded. From that point forward, when new cells are born, they contain that new genetic coding (a little like how the radioactive spider changes the DNA in Spider-Man). This recoding of the RNA allows scientists to then use a radioactive dye that will only attach to cells that have that new genetic coding, cells that were born after the radiation treatment. Scientists used that dye to look for new cells in brain tissue, and they discovered these new cells in and around the hippocampus, but nowhere else (Eriksson et al. 1998). Some of the people who donated their brains for this study were well into their eighties when they received the radiation treatment, suggesting that we grow these new brain cells throughout our entire life span. Amazing, right?

We call this process of growing new brain cells "neurogenesis." I think it's one of the coolest discoveries about the brain in the last century. I hope Dr. Eriksson and his team get the Nobel Prize. What's more, we have since learned that the growth of these brain cells isn't a passive phenomenon. You can jump in and exert control over the process, which I will teach you more about as you proceed through this workbook.

WOPR: Neurogenesis

Write. What is neurogenesis? How did we find it? (Paraphrase; put in your own words.)

_____

_____

_____

Quick quiz. Do new brain cells grow all over the brain? _____

Organize. Put your definition into a few bullet points.

- _____

- _____

- _____

Picture. Draw a picture related to neurogenesis.

_____

Rehearse. Practice over and over either your bullet points or your picture, or even picture your bullet points.

2. Cells Rewire

Brain plasticity is not all about growing new brain cells. Brain cells only grow in one small part of the brain and don't replenish themselves. If neurogenesis were the full story of brain plasticity, then I really don't think we would be this excited. Another important part of the story is that the brain cells you've had your whole life also grow and change based on how you use them.

Cells That Fire Together Wire Together

Way back in the 1930s and 1940s, a scientist named Donald Hebb demonstrated that neurons and nerve cells can rewire when they are stimulated in synchrony (made to fire together). We now call this "Hebb's law," which essentially states that *cells that fire together wire together.* Any type of nerve impulse or brain activity creates an electrical charge (firing), and when nerves and neurons fire at the same time, they wire up with one another. Hebb's law therefore explains that how you use your brain determines how your brain is wired (continuing throughout your entire life).

Why then, you might ask, are we calling this a new way of thinking about the brain, since we knew about this way back in the 1940s? Good question. You might not know this, but science can be political. The career path of most scientists involves climbing through the ranks of power, with one of the highest peaks becoming the editor of a scientific journal. You don't get the honor of becoming editor without some political clout. All the "buddy-buddy" stuff can lead to a culture of "groupthink," wherein many innovative ideas are discounted or ignored, especially if something new challenges the status quo and the work of your buddies.

After World War II, the field of neuroscience flourished. This was the era when IQ and cognitive testing were developed. Throughout this time, scientists were consumed with locating specific skills within specific regions of the brain. Thus, they couldn't, or wouldn't, entertain the idea that the brain could remold or rewire itself. It blew their minds, "did not compute," so the newly budding field of brain plasticity, spurred by Dr. Hebb, went into the dark ages for over four decades.

Norman Doidge (2007) provides an eloquent account of this epic battle between what he dubs the "locationists" (the dominating scientists dedicated to understanding which parts of the brain were responsible for which function) and those challenging this notion in his book *The Brain That Changes Itself.* This book also includes astonishing and inspiring examples of people remolding their brains and making incredible recoveries from strokes and other conditions.

High-powered journal editors refused to publish studies that used the term "brain plasticity" until another pioneer, Michael Merzenich came along in the mid-1980s. Dr. Merzenich showed evidence of brain cells rewiring that was so convincing the editors could no longer refuse to publish papers including the term "plasticity." He did this by mapping out which single brain cells responded to each finger on a monkey's hand and then looked at what happened to the activity of those brain cells when he removed the nerve input to the brain. At first the brain cells that lost the input stopped firing, but over time they came back online, responding to stimulation given to neighboring fingers (Merzenich et al. 1984).

These studies spurred a major shift in neuroscience. We have since learned how this rewiring process happens, which is through cells growing more synapses and connections getting stronger.

The Mechanics of Cells Rewiring

There are a few ways in which cells rewire (Nicoll 2017).

1. **Increased synaptic density.** The neurons you've had your whole life can grow more connections between each other, a process called increased synaptic density. They do this by growing new receiving branches (called dendrites) to reach out and connect to more neurons. This is sort of like business networking wherein you work to build your contacts and form new connections.

2. **Synaptogenesis.** At the end of these branches, the neuron can also grow more connection points (called synapses); this is called synaptogenesis.

3. **Long-term potentiation (LTP).** At the site of a specific synapse, the receiving cell will remold itself, so it can be more responsive to the cells sending it signals, a process called long-term potentiation (LTP). It will literally grow more receptor sites to increase the avenues through which the other cells can contact it. This is sort of like making a new friend. At first you trade phone numbers and start texting, and then as you get more acquainted, you connect on Facebook and so on.

Plasticity does go in both directions though, so if a pathway or connection is not being used, the connections will diminish. Use it or lose it is a thing. At the synapse itself, this is called long-term depression (LTD, the opposite of LTP); the receiving cell takes back the new receptor site if the cells stop communicating. This is sort of like muting or unfriending someone on Facebook you haven't seen or talked to in a while.

The use of the word "depression" here isn't the same as clinical depression or low mood. It's more neuroscience speak for "the opposite of potentiation," a withering away. However, we do know that LTD can be accelerated by clinical depression (Andrade and Kumar Rao 2010), so it is important to address this as well.

WOPR: Cells Rewiring

Write. How do brain cells rewire? (Paraphrase; put in your own words.)

_____

_____

_____

_____

_____

_____

Organize. Put your definition into a few bullet points.

- _____

- _____

- _____

Picture. Draw a picture related to cells rewiring.

Rehearse. Practice over and over either your bullet points or your picture, or even picture your bullet points.

3. Brain Regions Take on New Jobs

With advancing brain-scanning technology, we are able to watch activity change all over the brain as people learn new skills. For example, if you're learning a new skill, like swinging a golf club, during the process of learning, you are activating your prefrontal cortex because you are thinking, analyzing, and trying to remember. But as your skill advances, your overall brain activity actually goes down, not up. That is because the activity moves from your giant prefrontal cortex and into your basal ganglia, the site of your procedural memory in the middle of your brain, which is more efficient and requires less activity overall (Doyon and Benali 2005).

We are also able to watch regions of the brain take on entirely new jobs. In the late 1990s, a group of researchers wanted to see what parts of the brain were activated when they stimulated the fingertips of people who were born blind and could read Braille (Sadato et al. 1996). Some of the results were what they expected. The fingertip areas on the "somatosensory cortex" (the section of the outer covering of your brain that decodes physical sensations coming in through your body), which the locationists had identified decades before, were activated. But surprisingly some other parts of the brain were activated as well. The biggest surprise was that there was activity in the occipital lobe (at the back of the brain), because this region was previously thought to be entirely devoted to decoding input from your eyeballs and nothing else. This study proved that a region of the brain thought to be hardwired to the eyeballs was now being activated by input from the fingertips, meaning it had taken on a new job by virtue of the person learning Braille, a job that was never thought possible before we understood that the brain could rewire.

4. Brain Regions and Pathways Get Bigger

One of the first studies to show that brain regions get bigger through learning examined an elite group of taxi drivers in London. In the 1990s, a group of researchers wondered if there might be something different about the brains of these drivers, who must complete a three-to-four-year apprenticeship process to acquire what they literally call "the knowledge." It is so rigorous that 75 percent of the people who sign up for the apprenticeship drop out. The knowledge is the fastest way to get from point A to point B in the crazy maze of streets in central London.

The researchers compared MRI brain scans of the taxi drivers, bus drivers who followed a predetermined route, and regular drivers who drove themselves. They measured the size of various structures in the brains and found that the back tip of the hippocampus, a region thought to be associated with spatial memory, was bigger in the cab drivers.

You might think—and this is a good criticism—*Well, it's possible the cab drivers were just born that way*, which is what most people believed in the heyday of genetics; *having that part of the brain bigger was the trait that allowed the people to succeed in the training program.* So, the researchers were smart, and they followed a class of new recruits, measuring their brains before and after the three-to-four-year apprenticeship (Woolett and Maguire 2011). In people who had either not signed up for the apprenticeship or had dropped out, the back part of the hippocampus stayed the same size, but in the people who completed the apprenticeship, this back region of the hippocampus grew by about 30 percent. This provided some of the first evidence to show that brains were growing and changing based on experience.

Now you don't have to quit your job and move to London to become one of these cab drivers to increase the size of your brain, although a lot of people did consider doing this around 2011. Fortunately, we've since learned that similar growth happens every time you master a new skill, and it can happen much faster. We've seen evidence of connection pathways between regions of the brain (specifically, in and out of the front part of the brain) growing after practicing a visual memory-training technique for just eight weeks (Engvig et al. 2012).

Based on this evidence, by practicing the memory skills and exercises in this book, you can grow your brain as well, which will not only help you increase your investment in your brain 401(k) and lower your risk for dementia down the line, but you will also benefit in the short run by performing better at work, being a more attentive parent, or meeting any of those other goals you laid out at the beginning of the book.

WOPR: Brain Regions Get Bigger and Take on New Jobs

Write. What did you learn about brain regions getting bigger, pathways growing through experience, and parts of the brain thought to be hardwired taking on entirely new jobs? (Be sure to paraphrase.)

_____

_____

_____

_____

_____

_____

Organize. Put your definition into a few bullet points.

- _____

- _____

- _____

Picture. Draw a picture related to brain regions getting bigger and taking on new jobs.

Rehearse. Practice over and over either your bullet points or your picture, or even picture your bullet points.

Cognitive Control Network

Here's the thing. You can't really expect your brain to change if you're lying on the couch playing Candy Crush. Functional brain imaging research has revealed two brain networks that are consistently activated: one when engaged in a task (cognitive control network) and the other when "resting" or "disengaging" (default mode network).

The default mode network (DMN; Raichle et al. 2001) seems to be responsible for brain activity related to daydreaming and thinking about yourself, the mode that you would expect your mind to go into if you were lying inside an MRI tube and told to "do nothing." You can imagine what this feels like, right? I like to describe it as being kind of "back," like how you would lean back or look up when daydreaming. Also, most of the structures involved in the DMN are farther back in your brain.

Take a moment to daydream and "do nothing" and jot down some notes of what the DMN "feels" like to you.

_____

_____

_____

The cognitive control network (CCN; Niendam et al. 2012) is more forward, involving more of your frontal lobes. It involves focusing, concentration, and engagement. Also, think about how you sit and look when you're engaged in something; you probably tend to lean forward.

You've probably been in CCN for most of this chapter. Take a moment to jot down some notes of what this network "feels" like to you.

_____

_____

_____

It doesn't seem that a whole lot of positive brain plasticity takes place in the default mode except maybe some memory rehearsal and visioning for the future. Typically, in DMN, you're running old scripts and doing habitual things, like lining up the four red candies to make a striped candy, unless you're visioning for your future (Schacter et al. 2012).

Engaging the cognitive control network, though, seems to promote the most positive brain plasticity. For many decades, before we even knew about these networks, evidence was mounting that engagement is key for growing new brain pathways and changing your brain. Engaging and focusing seems to provide the novelty and challenge needed to help you mold new pathways and change your brain (Han, Chapman, and Krawczyk 2018).

Dose-Response Curve

There really aren't any hard-and-fast rules yet on how much practice of a new skill you need to change your brain. We have seen documented brain changes where people practiced a new skill for as little as a twenty-five minutes per day, five days per week for eight weeks (Engvig et al. 2012). Some media reports tout brain changes that happen faster with less practice. Here's the thing: There are so many factors that play into all of this. For one, we know that physical activity can rapidly accelerate this process (Gradari et al. 2016), as well as age, type of information, prior experience, hormones—all sorts of stuff (White et al. 2013). Plus, then there is the whole thing about it taking ten thousand hours of practice to become an expert at something (Gladwell 2008).

Also keep in mind that plasticity isn't a static process. It is incredibly dynamic. Again, use it or lose it is a thing. Keeping pathways active so they don't wither also makes a difference.

A lot of the dose-response curve also depends on what you're trying to rewire. In treating clinical depression, we are starting to use neuroplasticity to explain what happens in psychotherapy. By teaching people to limit self-defeating thoughts and behaviors and helping them shift to more supportive thoughts, we have been rewiring their brains for decades. But people respond to these interventions quite differently, and one factor is how deeply entrenched those old limiting beliefs are. A well-worn path is likely harder to rewire than some novel idea. All of these factors make it hard to nail down a precise dose-response curve for plasticity. What we do know though is that plasticity rarely happens with one dose, so practice is key.

Now that you know that your brain can remold itself based on how you use it, let's harness this knowledge and let the brain training begin! In the next part of the book, "The Skills," I will guide you through a neuroscience-based roadmap for building the best memory of your life.

Part II

The Skills

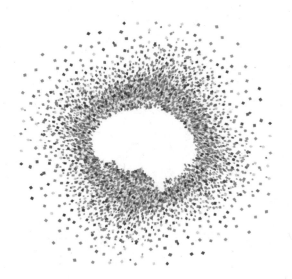

Chapter 6

Move Your Body to Build a Bigger Brain

It is no secret that being more active is good for you. I'm sure this comes as no shock to you. Physical activity (or the dreaded word "exercise"—yikes!) is frequently called the most effective, most commonly available, and most underutilized panacea for practically every ailment from heart disease to diabetes to depression to, yes, memory. And yet, far too many of us don't do nearly enough of it. Why? We resist, we resist, we resist.

This chapter is about how physical activity can help your brain and your memory. I will present some of the exciting new research that shows how moving your body helps your brain.

I do not want to pile on you a bunch of "shoulds." I don't want you to feel ashamed of your activity level because shame is immobilizing. I want to inspire you, and once you know how incredibly beneficial moving your body is for your memory, and we remove some of your mental roadblocks, I think you'll be out there boppin' along, movin' around like never before.

Listen, I get the resistance. There are definitely times when I fall off my physical activity routine and find myself being way too sedentary. The downside is not just physical but also mental. I get grumpy and foggy, lose things, and even struggle with conversations a bit now that I'm in my forties. When I admit that I'm in one of those stages, I use the exercises below to try and pop myself out of it. My aim here is to help you build up the motivation, courage, and support you need to get your body moving, while also soaking in all of the brain (and body) benefits. But first, let's get a sense of what's been holding you back.

Reasons I Hate/Can't Do Exercise

Now let's talk about resistance. We all have reasons for why we don't move more, whether it's asthma, paralysis, chronic pain, a bum knee, or just good-old mental resistance. Use the lines on the following page to list all the reasons why you don't exercise regularly. I've provided some categories to help stimulate "reasons" in case you get stuck.

You might discover through this exercise that some of these "reasons" are actually automatic, self-defeating thoughts like *I don't have the energy*, or *People will stare at my butt at the gym*. Don't censor yourself here. Don't judge. We all have these thoughts. It's important that you capture these thoughts. Why? You may think it's counterproductive to expose yourself to such negativity, but it's essential that you get access to these negative thoughts because you are generating these thoughts already. When you don't capture them, they have tremendous power over you. Your brain automatically accepts them as 100 percent true, but if you capture them, then you can have power over them. You get a choice in how much you accept them to be true, which I'm betting in most cases is less than 100 percent, and that is a tremendous improvement.

My "Reasons" for Not Being More Physically Active

Initial "reasons" (list the first things that come to mind, like "I don't have time"):

_____   _____

_____   _____

Physical "reasons" (for example, asthma, bum knee, heart problem):

_____   _____

_____   _____

Identity "reasons" (for example, "Exercise is for skinny people and meatheads," "Exercise might trigger my eating disorder," or "I don't fit at the gym"):

_____   _____

_____   _____

Lack of success (for example, "I never stick with it," "I never get anywhere," "I always quit," or "I'm not motivated"):

_____   _____

_____   _____

The Science: Why Physical Activity Is Likely the Best Thing You Can Do for Your Brain

One great way to get motivated is to understand the science. From a neuroscience perspective, moving your body seems to be the best way to improve your memory and brain. We have solid experimental evidence in both animals and humans to show that when you are physically active, many positive things happen in your brain. Physical activity helps you build a bigger (yes, I said bigger), stronger brain and a stronger memory. Here are seven ways that physical activity helps your brain and memory.

1. What's Good for Your Heart Is Good for Your Brain

Early in the days of understanding cognitive reserve, or brain 401(k), physical activity was one of the first lifestyle behaviors to be linked to people with bigger brains. At first, scientists did not fully understand the link, and initially many assumed that the brain benefits were related to the well-known cardiovascular benefits of exercise. What's good for your heart is good for your brain, and this is still very much the case. Your brain is very reliant on your heart. Brain cells require steady blood flow to stay alive because they cannot store their own energy. You can cut off circulation to your arm and be all right for a while, but if you do not get blood flow to your brain, cells start dying within a matter of three to five minutes. Therefore, it stands to reason that engaging in physical activity and strengthening your heart and vascular system provides important benefits to your brain, and this is true.

2. Grow More Blood Vessels

We've been talking a lot about the plasticity of the brain, but did you know that your vasculature is also plastic (changeable)? When you're more physically active, you're pumping blood to the ends of your vasculature, and as a result, you grow more blood vessels, particularly down in the capillary tips of your blood vessels. This broadens the blood supply to your brain, because more vessels are feeding it, delivering more of the oxygen and sugar your brain cells need to work and stay alive. This expansion of the vasculature also comes in handy if a small artery feeding blood to the brain gets blocked by a blood clot or some plaque in your arteries (a stroke). By being more physically active and growing more blood vessel branches, the cells fed by that blocked artery have a better chance of staying alive because by exercising you have grown a "back door" supply of blood flow that wouldn't have been there otherwise.

3. Grow More Brain Cells

Being physically active helps you grow more of those new brain cells we talked about in chapter 5. As you may recall, *adults grow new brain cells*, a process we call "neurogenesis." But keep in mind that you don't grow a lot of them, so you need to keep the ones you have. But what's even more exciting is that you can control and help this process by moving your body. Growing more brain cells is especially important for memory because, as you might also recall, these new brain cells only grow in and around the major memory center in your brain, the hippocampus (figure 7). Thus, they seem to play a big role in helping you form new long-term memories. So, if you want to give yourself a memory boost, move your body to grow more brain cells in the explicit memory center of your brain.

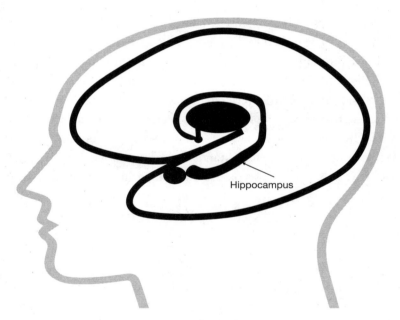

Figure 7. Neurogenesis—the growth of new brain cells in adulthood—within the brain only occurs in and around the hippocampus. People who are more physically active grow more of these new neurons.

4. Increase Nerve Growth Factors

In addition to growing more brain cells when you bike, jog, walk, swim, or whatever, we also know that your body produces some very important chemicals that are used in the growth and rewiring of your brain cells. These chemicals are called "nerve growth factors." Many people have described them as Miracle-Gro for your brain cells. Without these chemicals, cells in the brain and body do not grow. They are proteins that help with the type of "signaling" that cells must do to grow and change. They help stimulate the growth of new brain cells and help your new baby brain cells grow up to become new neurons by turning on the "grow up" signals that are needed for this process. They also help the brain cells you have had your whole life do the rewiring activities I described in chapter 5, signaling the cells to grow new synapses, or connections with one another.

There are many different types of these nerve growth factors. Two get the most attention: brain-derived neurotrophic factor (BNDF) is part of a class of chemicals called neurotrophins that do a lot of the growth signaling described above, and insulin-like growth factor 1 (IGF-1) works with human growth hormone to literally build your body and brain. We thought for a while that cardio activities led to increased production of BDNF, while strength training promoted IFG-1, but the jury may still be out on this one. At any rate, it seems that the best approach with exercise is to do what doctors have been telling us for decades, which is to do a variety of both cardio and strengthening activities, regularly.

5. Build a Bigger Brain

Another exciting benefit to physical activity is that it can give you a bigger brain (Erickson, Leckie, and Weinstein 2014; Neth et al. 2020). Longitudinal studies (where people are followed over time; Erickson et al. 2010) show that older adults who walk at least one mile per day have more gray matter (a plumper collection of the cell bodies of neurons) in important areas like the prefrontal cortex (the place where you organize information to remember it better). We also have solid experimental evidence, in humans, showing that vigorous activity grows the hippocampus, the star of our show (Erickson et al. 2011). Experimental evidence is the best kind of evidence because it allows us to say that one thing caused another: in this case exercise caused a bigger hippocampus.

This finding, that exercise leads to a bigger brain, deserves a story. About a decade ago, scientists performed a study where they evenly divided a group of women in their sixties into two groups for an exercise program (Erickson et al. 2011). The two groups completed an hour-long exercise program, three times a week for a year. One group performed stretching and toning exercises, while the other group engaged in a vigorous walking class where they basically marched in place for an hour in what added up to about a two-mile walk. The researchers measured the size of the ladies' hippocampi (plural for "hippocampus") to see what happened over the course of the year. What they found was that in the stretching and toning group, the hippocampus shrunk by about 1.5 percent, which is the normal rate of shrinkage for women that age (that, in and of itself, is depressing), but the good news is that in the vigorous walking group, the hippocampus *grew* by 2 percent.

The study authors concluded that vigorous activity "reverses one to two years of age-related [brain] volume loss," a conclusion that I find to be so inspiring. Moving your body is free for the taking. Maybe you have to buy yourself a new pair of sneakers, but otherwise, what's stopping you?

Quick caveat: While it is important to keep up your physical activity routine, the plumping up of the hippocampus is most dramatic during that "couch to 5K" phase. People who are already pretty physically active when they start these types of experiments do not show these dramatic effects, seemingly because their hippocampi are already plump. Furthermore, there is still a lot for us to learn about the how and the why behind all of these brain-growth changes. We still really aren't sure of the exact mechanisms behind increasing gray matter. In most parts of the brain, the growth is *not* because you're getting more brain cells, since they only grow in and around the hippocampus. Our best guess at this point is that the nerve growth factors that are increased by physical activity are allowing the brain cells you've had your whole life to get bigger by growing more connection branches (specifically more dendrites, sprouting more dendritic branches, like a bush or a tree).

6. Activate Your Relaxation Response

You will learn more about the role of stress in your brain and memory later on. For now, let me just tell you that the opposite of the "fight-or-flight response" (the body sensations you feel when you are scared or angry) is what we call "rest-and-digest." It's a state of calm, and in most cases, this results in better focus in the present moment and better memory down the line.

When you are physically active, say running or walking quickly, your body is in the fight-or-flight state. This is good. You are burning off the stress hormones and putting your stress response to the purpose nature intended: running away from a predator. Worrying does not do this; it makes you pump out more stress hormones. The coolest part of physical activity is that when you are finished running or walking or whatever you did to get your heart rate up, your body automatically goes into the rest-and-digest state, allowing you to be calm and focused. This is the same state you feel after you've meditated or had a really amazing massage. Along with the endorphins (morphine or opioids that your body produces) you get with exercise, this rest-and-digest rebound is a big part of why exercise feels so good when you're done.

7. Remember Stuff Better Now

And finally, the result you've been waiting for. Isn't having a better memory now one of the main reasons you're reading this book? Well physical activity does that for you too. I know I'm starting to sound like an infomercial: *"But wait! There's more."* But I'm not making this stuff up. Experiments show that if you exercise before you learn something new, you will remember it better. Likely because your brain is primed for the learning. You've cranked out a new baby brain cell or two, and you've flooded your brain with nerve growth factors, so bring on the memory.

These seven reasons convinced me to believe that being more physically active is likely the very best thing we can do for our brain and our memory (Sng, Frith, and Loprinzi 2018). So, here is my rule of thumb. When you're considering whether or not to invest your time, money, and energy into a brain fitness activity like crosswords or online brain games, ask yourself, *Am I doing this at the expense of moving my body?* I know we all experience avoidance. Believe me, I'm right there with you. I do things at the expense of moving my body all the time, but this question is a big part of what keeps me motivated to move my body as often as I can.

Try the Memory Challenge Yourself

This exercise requires you to be ready to move your body and to have a timer. You could use the clock app on your phone.

Below are two different grocery lists. You will study each list for one minute and then write the items from memory in the spaces next to them (obviously you'll need to cover the list with your hand, some paper, or your coffee mug so you're not cheating). You don't have to write the items in the same order; just write as many as you can. The only difference between the first list and the second list is that you will memorize and recall the first list before you do fifteen (or more) minutes of some activity (a fitness video, a walk, marching in place, your normal run or water aerobics class, and so forth), and you will do the second list after your workout.

List 1: Get Your Sneakers On, but Do This First

Got your sneakers on? Okay, so before you move your body, study this list of words for only one minute—set a timer. Then when the timer goes off, cover the list and write as many words as you can remember. Don't cheat by peaking after your first recall. Be honest with yourself.

Bananas   _____

Oranges   _____

Green beans   _____

Salmon   _____

Couscous   _____

Bread   _____

Swiss cheese   _____

Birthday cake   _____

List 2: Learn While You're Sweaty

Okay, so now that you've been active, try the memory challenge again with the list below. Like before, study this list of words for only one minute—set a timer. When the timer goes off, cover the list and write as many words as you can remember. Don't cheat. Be honest with yourself.

Apples   _____

Grapes   _____

Salad greens   _____

Chicken   _____

Brown rice   _____

Bagels   _____

Cheddar cheese   _____

Cookies   _____

How did it go? Did you notice any difference?

_____

_____

_____

_____

The Benefits of Physical Activity

Now that you've had a chance to learn more about the science, take some time to check all the benefits of being more physically active that apply to you.

- ☐ More energy
- ☐ Trimmer waistline
- ☐ Stronger muscles
- ☐ Better posture
- ☐ Lower blood sugar
- ☐ Lower blood pressure
- ☐ More confidence
- ☐ A better mood
- ☐ Being nicer to my friends and family
- ☐ A stronger heart
- ☐ Stronger lungs
- ☐ A bigger brain
- ☐ More oxygen to my brain
- ☐ Grow more brain cells
- ☐ Release endorphins (natural morphine)
- ☐ Handle stress better
- ☐ Reduce the impact of stress on my body
- ☐ Look better in my clothes

- ☐ Increased cognitive reserve
- ☐ Wearing "those jeans" again
- ☐ Being more active with kids
- ☐ Staying more mobile
- ☐ Staying more independent
- ☐ Reducing disabilities
- ☐ Releasing muscle tension
- ☐ Calming my worries
- ☐ Having fun things to do with friends
- ☐ Being part of a team
- ☐ Lower risk for dementia
- ☐ Learn something new (like ping-pong, dance, better walking stride)
- ☐ Reduced fall risk (this protects your noggin)
- ☐ Feeling good about taking care of myself
- ☐ A better memory

New Reasons Why I Want to Be More Physically Active

Now, I want you to distill the list of benefits to your top three to five reasons for why you want to be more physically active. These are your "whys," and it is important to *keep your why close by*. For that reason, I want you to write your whys twice: once here in the book, and again on a piece of paper that you can post in a place you will see it often. This will become your "can't miss reminder." Tape it to your bathroom mirror or above your coffee pot, any place you will see it on a daily basis. Plus writing it twice equals repetition, another important memory strategy.

My Whys

_____

_____

_____

_____

_____

What Activities Do You Enjoy?

What physical activities do you enjoy? You may be thinking, *None*, and that's okay. A good way to get started is by thinking about activities you enjoyed in the past, maybe even in the distant past, like when you were a kid. I understand it's not always feasible to do the things you did as a kid, but it could serve as a good starting point in your brainstorming. For example, if you loved running as a kid, you could go on long walks. If you were a gymnast, dancer, or cheerleader, you could turn on some disco music and bop around your living room.

If you have a physical disability, keep in mind that being more physically active is often feasible, you may just need to get some help from a physical therapist. They can help you modify your activity so it's safe and achievable and help you acquire modified equipment, such as a three-wheel recumbent bike or in-home exercise machines.

The main goal of the next exercise is to be completely open to the joy that comes from certain activities. Don't judge or censor yourself as you work through the checklist and brainstorming spaces. Try to connect to your desire and joy so you can figure out ways to be more physically active to help your memory.

I've listed some ideas to get you started. This list is by no means exhaustive, so if some things you enjoy or enjoyed in the past are not on the list, write them in the spaces below.

Activities That You Enjoy Now or Enjoyed in the Past

Check all that apply to you.

☐ Swimming	☐ Basketball	☐ Running around on a playground
☐ Biking	☐ Yoga	☐ Swinging
☐ Running	☐ Tai chi	☐ Jump rope
☐ Walking	☐ Wrestling	☐ Boxing
☐ Dancing	☐ Lifting weights	☐ Pilates
☐ Bowling	☐ Circuit training	☐ Tennis/handball/squash/pickleball
☐ Soccer	☐ Aerobics	☐ Ping-pong/table tennis
☐ Football	☐ Elliptical machine	☐ Boccie ball
☐ Cheerleading	☐ StairMaster	☐ Pool/billiards
☐ Volleyball	☐ Lunges and squats	
☐ Softball/baseball	☐ Sit-ups/crunches	

Other:

_____   _____   _____

_____   _____   _____

_____   _____   _____

How Much Exercise Do You Need?

People ask me all the time, "How much physical activity do I need to do then?" Based on what we know so far, there does not seem to be a point of diminishing returns when it comes to physical activity's benefits to the brain. The more you do, the better. Marathon runners seem to reap a lot of brain benefits, particularly with respect to cranking out those new brain cells. But please *do not hurt yourself.* Please don't take this fact to mean that you have to start running marathons, unless you just really want to and you're able. You don't have to exercise to the extreme, because every little bit counts.

In terms of protecting yourself from dementia, consider walking six to nine mile per week, provided you are able, an important baseline for your physical activity (Erickson et al. 2010). In a study of people in their seventies who were followed over nine years, those who walked six to nine miles per week (seventy-two blocks) were less likely to develop dementia during that period of time (they also had bigger brains). You could also use the general recommendation of at least ten thousand steps a day as a baseline, and then monitor yourself with a pedometer, like a Fitbit.

If you have a physical disability that prevents you from reaching these benchmarks, I recommend you see a physical therapist and ask them to give you a group of exercises that you can do to get your heart pumping. I'm confident this can help, and it's likely that insurance will cover it. Greater physical activity is achievable at every age, with every body size, and with every ability level.

Goals

It's a good idea to set some physical activity goals, but a goal without a plan is a wish. Next, you are going to set a few goals, starting with your long-range goals down to your "no-big-deal, get-started" step. This will help you create a plan. *(You can also download a printable copy of this exercise at http:// newharbinger.com/47438.)*

Long-Range Goals

This is more like a vision. Close your eyes for a minute and think about yourself twenty to thirty years from now. (If you're already eighty or ninety, then you can shave off a couple of years from this vision, if you want.) Imagine you have kept the same lifestyle habits you have now over the past two to three decades. What do you look like? What are you doing? How well are you getting around? How is your memory?

Cindy wrote: Oh man, I do not like what I see. I'll be almost as old as my mom is now, and I'm not sure I'm aging as well as she did. She used to walk every day. My brain is going to go to total mush if I don't do something soon, plus I'll be all slumped over.

Write some notes here of what your vision looks like.

_____

_____

_____

_____

If this vision isn't so positive, then let's tweak it a little bit. What do you want it to look like? What do you want to be doing? Imagine the best possible outcome. You're energized. You're able. You're remembering things.

Cindy wrote: **If I start walking a few times a week, I may have more energy, and my brain may work better. I'll go for that promotion at work, so maybe I can retire a little earlier and play golf.**

Jot down some notes about your revised vision.

_____

_____

_____

_____

What do you need to start doing now to move toward this second vision and away from the first?

Cindy wrote: **New sneakers, a plan; I'll put walk times in my calendar, look into yoga classes, and maybe golf lessons.**

Jot down your ideas.

_____

_____

_____

_____

Excellent. This vision is an important first step for your plan. Now we need to start thinking about some action steps, and it also helps to set some midrange goals. These benchmarks help you move along your journey. Also, if you're the type who needs a reward (a carrot), then make sure to write down some rewards for yourself for achieving these shorter and midrange goals. Sometimes achieving the goals is reward enough, but that's not the case for everyone.

Midrange Goals

Whether it's to complete a charity 5K, like the Walk to End Alzheimer's; dance at a wedding; or show off some new muscles, it helps to have some midrange goals to keep you motivated. You might think of these as "carrots" as you lead your "turtle-self" to moving your body. Also make sure to jot down the reward—it could be the T-shirt from the charity race, the pictures from the wedding, or even a more tangible reward, like chocolate or money.

"In six to twelve months, I want to be able to..."

Cindy wrote: **Get through a whole yoga class doing most of the moves, and be able to play nine holes of golf and have fun.**

Your goal: _____

_____

_____

_____

Cindy's reward: **That new putter I've been eyeing online.**

Your reward: _____

_____

_____

Shorter-Term Goals

It can be really hard to stay motivated if your only "carrot" is six to twelve months away, so go ahead and jot down some shorter-term goals for the next month or two. These are some short-range steps to get you to your midrange and long-term goals, like working up to walking a particular distance, checking off a particular number of days when you do your activity, and so forth. Identify a reward for yourself, too, while you're at it; it doesn't have to be fancy, just motivating.

"In one to two months, I want to be able to…"

Cindy wrote: **Make it to yoga class without dreading it and log three walks a week like it's normal.**

Your goal: _____

_____

_____

Cindy's reward: **A new yoga outfit.**

Your reward: _____

_____

_____

The No-Big-Deal, Get-Started Step

The biggest pitfall of goal setting is that goals are often too lofty, so people lose motivation very quickly. So now is your chance to just get yourself started. I call this the "no-big-deal, get-started step." What is the first small step you need to take toward your short-term goal? Whatever that one step is, ask yourself, *Can I do it with no resistance?* If not, cut it in half. If you can't do that without resistance, cut it in half again. Keep cutting in half until you get to your "no-big-deal, get-started step." That's when you say to yourself, *Oh, that's no big deal. I can do that.*

"I will do this no-big-deal, get-started step to move me toward my goal either right now or later today or tomorrow..."

Cindy wrote: **I will lay my sneakers and my walking clothes next to my bed.**

Your no-big-deal, get-started step: _____

_____

Get Yourself Some Support

You don't have to do all of this alone. In fact, you're more likely to be successful if you engage some allies in your activity journey (any journey really, but let's focus on the task at hand). If you've already experienced some declines, then this next step is likely even more crucial, since you may already have people looking out for you. It's understandable if you're feeling timid about asking for help, especially if you feel that others are doing a lot for you already, but I want you to push yourself to do this.

Your Cheering Squad

In the spaces below on the left, write the names of some people who can support you as you increase your physical activity and on the right side, write down the specific action you'd like them to take on your behalf. For example, if you need to hire a personal trainer or start physical therapy, write the trainer or therapist's name on the left (you can write the company name or "trainer" for now if you don't yet know one personally) and then the action on the right, such as "guide me through exercises three times a week." If you want to start walking more and you know your friend or neighbor might be willing to be your walking buddy, put her name down on the left and "walk around the neighborhood Monday and Friday mornings" on the right. It's brainstorming, so you do not have to have all of the details yet, but try to be as specific as possible. You are setting an intention. It doesn't have to be perfect, but with any intention details help.

Name of Person to Help You Move More	What This Person Will Do

I imagine you may have never considered physical activity to be the first of many strategies to improve your memory. I hope by now that the reason it is number one on the list is clear. This understanding may provide more motivation to increase your activity. If you still struggle with motivation, that's understandable. Perhaps by practicing some of the exercises in this chapter, the motivation will continue to build. Now let's move on to explore even more ways to improve your memory.

Chapter 7

Learn New Things

The second skill for building a better memory is to learn new things. It flows nicely after moving your body because it is an important "part 2" to the growing new brain cells story. In this chapter, I'll teach you the neuroscience of why learning new things is so critical to building a better memory, along with some strategies to make it easier to learn new things.

The Science Behind Learning New Things

Remember those baby brain cells you just grew on your walk? Well those are not instantly new neurons. These baby brain cells start off as stem cells, those magical cells that can become any cell in the body (Gould et al. 2000). To become a new neuron, the stem cells must be "trained" and given a job. This means they have to be stimulated by existing, neighboring neurons to become a new neuron themselves. Don't forget, new brain cells only grow in and around the hippocampus, not all over the brain, and the hippocampus is where you encode your new explicit, long-term memories for facts and events. Therefore, to stimulate these baby brain cells, what do you need to do? You need to use your hippocampus, fire it up, get it active by making new memories and learning something new. Or else they die…

If no firing or memory making happens, if these stem cells aren't stimulated, trained, and given a job, then the baby brain cells get "reabsorbed by the system" (Gould et al. 2000). This is just a nice way of saying they die. So, if you want the new baby brain cells you birthed while dancing, swimming, or running to stick around and help you out, it's best that you also spend some time learning new things. If you're doing the same old thing all the time, then you're not stimulating the hippocampus or the new stem cells in the same way. Once new things become old habits, the brain activity moves out of the hippocampal part of the brain to the basal ganglia where no new brain cells grow (Poldrack et al. 2001).

Let's check in. I just laid some serious neuroscience on you. How are you taking it in? Write some thoughts and reactions here.

_____

_____

_____

More Than Just Brain Games

In the early studies of cognitive reserve, intellectual engagement, along with physical and social activity, was one of the top predictors of higher reserve. This finding launched the field of "brain fitness" in the early 2000s. A whole new industry of software companies, like Lumosity and Posit Science, sprung to life, propelled by intense fears of Alzheimer's. I got involved in the brain fitness field early on, but I quickly noticed that a lot was lacking. Many important elements of brain health were being overlooked in the search for "silver bullets" or "magic pills" (Marx 2013), which a lot of people thought were these brain games.

I don't intend to criticize brain fitness efforts, but you should know that the early marketing claims of brain fitness products rapidly outpaced the research. Companies touted their brain games to prevent dementia without proof. Lumosity was fined by the Federal Trade Commission in 2016 for false advertising (Underwood 2016), and subsequent scientific reviews have shown that brain-training software has limited effectiveness in preventing dementia (Livingston et al. 2017). I don't think there is a lot of harm in playing brain games unless you are playing them at the expense of moving your body and learning new things.

People often ask me, "Should I be doing sudoku or crossword puzzles?" My answer is, "It depends." The essential components of any brain-building activity are "*novelty, variety, and challenge*" (Fernandez and Goldberg 2009). *Novelty* provides much needed stimulation to the hippocampal region of the brain, where the new brain cells grow. *Variety* is important because you need all your brain skills to function day-to-day. If you only do crosswords (a verbal task) but nothing to stimulate the visual or math parts of your brain, then you're only building one skill (like only doing bicep curls with your left arm). And if you stay in your comfort zone and don't *challenge* yourself, then your brain will stay exactly the way it is and decline with age. If you do sudoku or brain games to zone out, fall asleep, or wind down, then I doubt they are helping you build reserve. The secret sauce is in learning a variety of new things that challenge you. You're doing it right now. You can also do it by taking a course, watching TED Talks, learning stories about your friends, studying music, traveling to new places, helping a kid with homework, trying out a new recipe, taking on a new healthy habit, and stuff like that.

The What: Make Your Brain Bucket List

What are some things you want to learn? I'm betting you have a list in your mind somewhere of things that you've always wanted to "dig into" or "learn about." Maybe you want to take a deep dive into some point in history or read classic literature. Maybe you want to learn interior design, a new language, how to knit, or how make a soufflé. Maybe your new thing is taking up the crossword because you never did it before, or if you're a crossword person and "not a numbers person," try your hand at sudoku. Maybe you want to take up a new physical activity, like golf, pickleball, or line dancing. If you worry that you don't have money for a new hobby, you could take a financial literacy class to build up your brain's "money management" pathway. As part of that process, you could save up for a trip abroad. Travel is a great way to learn new things, and it may provide the motivation you need to actually want to study another language.

Spend a few moments dreaming about your brain bucket list and write your ideas below. Whatever you pick, don't put things on here that you feel are shoulds. You're just not going to enjoy them. Nobody "has" to learn a new language to get a better brain. If something you pick has a tinge of "should" (for example, something you're not all that interested in but seems like a good idea), rephrase it as, "I want to," because ultimately it is a choice.

Your Brain Bucket List

The Why: Take Action to Learn New Things

Getting clear on why you want to do the things on your brain bucket list can help you feel more connected to the goal and increase your motivation.

Take Action on Your Brain Bucket List

Pick an item (or two) off your brain bucket list and follow this plan to implement it.

1. Brain bucket list item you chose: _____

2. Why you want to try this new activity. (Be specific and work in some feeling on this one. Does the activity help you connect to a fond memory—practicing Spanish to reminisce about that trip to Spain or Mexico—or help you connect to other people in your life, like a book club or cooking class?):

_____

_____

_____

_____

3. Benefits (what you expect to get out of learning this new thing): _____

_____

_____

4. What you need to get started (sign up for a class, take skydiving safety course, and so forth):

_____   _____

_____   _____

_____   _____

5. When you plan to try the new activity (Be specific—put it in your calendar.): _____

_____

_____

(You can download additional copies of this form at http://newharbinger.com/47438.)

The How: Encoding Strategies Make It Easier to Learn New Things

How you learn the new things on your brain bucket list can really vary. Sometimes learning is built into the item, such as taking a course. Other times the learning happens almost through osmosis, like through travel. Whatever the activity, learning new things can always be supported by knowing and practicing some basic memory strategies. Therefore, we are going to pivot a bit now and spend the rest of this chapter learning and practicing some additional memory strategies that will support you as you check off items on your brain bucket list.

In earlier chapters, you used a lot of WOPR to help you learn all that crazy neuroscience as we laid the foundation for this book's seven skills. Since WOPR is designed to help you more easily learn new things, I want to revisit WOPR and drill a few of the WOPR strategies to help you use it more fluently and efficiently in your daily life. Using WOPR to learn new things helps you train up your baby brain cells to become fully contributing members of your neuron society. WOPR is like college for your baby brain cells. My hope is that by using these memorization strategies, you will have more memory success in your daily life and check off items on your brain bucket list faster and more efficiently.

The drill (like basketball drills) involves memorizing some word lists with increasing use of WOPR-like strategies. (This exercise is from the cognitive rehabilitation program CogSMART, Twamley et al. 2012; the full ten-week program can be completed with a rehabilitation professional.) To start, memorize the first list using your existing skills.

Practice Learning Lists: List 1

Study the following list of words for one minute (set a timer). Then write them down from memory on a sheet of paper. Ready, go.

• Falcon	• Diamond	• Hawk	• Emerald
• Spark plug	• Hub cap	• Owl	• Oak
• Elm	• Pine	• Alternator	• Sapphire
• Eagle	• Maple	• Ruby	• Wheel

How many did you get? Write your total from list 1 here: _____

Excellent. Now let's see if we can improve your performance by adding in some WOPR strategies.

Pop Quiz Time

What does WOPR stand for, and how do you pronounce it?

WOPR sounds like: _____

WOPR stands for: W: _____ O: _____ P: _____ R: _____

If you don't remember all of the details of WOPR, that's okay. You can flip back to chapter 3 to refresh your memory. Also, don't feel bad. I hope you know by now that memory is not perfect.

Organize with Chunking

Organizing information helps your memory centers encode it better. "Chunking" is an effective organization strategy whereby you group information together into chunks, making smaller bits of information to be stored. Studies show that chunking in a systematized way can lead to all sorts of improvements in focus and memory, even for people with early stage Alzheimer's disease (Huntley et al. 2017). The acronym WOPR is a form of chunking because you're remembering four different concepts chunked into one word. Chunking can also be performed when memorizing lists of things, sometimes called categorizing.

"Categorizing" involves grouping words from a list based on some similar feature or category. It is a powerful strategy because it capitalizes on the natural way language is stored in your brain. Words are stored in what we call "semantic networks" (Bookheimer 2002). "Semantic" means "words and their meanings," so in a semantic network, words with similar features or in similar categories are linked together naturally in the brain. "Dog" is related to "cat," which is related to "mouse," which is related to "hamster," and so on. You can capitalize on this natural association when trying to remember new things by grouping similar items together. Then all you have to do is recall the category, which will cue you to think of the items within. This strategy works really well with shopping lists; for example, you can organize your grocery list according to department (produce, deli, and so forth) and aisle (baking, cereal, and so forth).

Practice Chunking Your Shopping List

Surely you need some stuff at the store. Spend a couple of moments brainstorming items that you need, and then you will go back and chunk them. Don't chunk yet; just brainstorm.

_____   _____

_____   _____

_____   _____

_____   _____

_____   _____

Now create some categories and organize your shopping list according to those groups, such as by aisle or section of the grocery store: produce, dairy, bakery, snacks, and so on.

Categories:

_____   _____   _____   _____

Items in each category:

_____   _____   _____   _____

_____   _____   _____   _____

_____   _____   _____   _____

_____   _____   _____   _____

_____   _____   _____   _____

Practice Learning Lists: List 2

Now it's time to memorize list 2 using your new O skills. As you read the following list of words, put them into categories below, and then write them down on a separate sheet of paper from memory.

Ready, go.

- Cat
- Carrot
- Broccoli
- Bread

- Mop
- Hose
- Asparagus
- Milk

- Sponge
- Eggs
- Vacuum
- Dog

- Bird
- Juice
- Hamster
- Onion

Category 1: _____

Category 2: _____

Category 3: _____

Category 4: _____

How many did you get? Write the total from list 2 here: _____

Make Visual Notes: Picture

You've had some experience with the picture step when you were making visual notes, but I want to add to your visualization skills and do some more drilling. Don't forget, visualization strategies are very powerful because they call upon your right Papez circuit, that other memory encoding system, in your right hemisphere, that you probably don't use as much as you could (because humans have evolved to prioritize reading, writing, and speaking).

Mental Snapshot

When you're in a pinch, under a time crunch to learn something new, a mental snapshot can be very handy. You can take mental snapshots of things, such as where you placed your keys, where you parked your car, or the contents of your refrigerator before you leave for the store. You do have to stop and pay attention, and then just snap a mental picture as though you're snapping a real photo. Your eyelids can be the "shutter." Look at the thing, snap the photo, close your eyes, and see it behind your eyelids.

Try it now. Take a mental snapshot of the table you're sitting at or the nearest side table. Look at the table; take a snapshot with your eyelids, see the items behind your eyelids, and list the items here:

_____   _____

_____   _____

_____   _____

Roman Room Method

Another widely used visualization strategy is the "method of loci" or the "journey method." I've also heard it called the "Roman room method" and the "memory palace" because it was used by ancient Romans, and likely the Greeks before them, as a strategy to remember epic tales before reading and writing were widespread.

We now have research showing that practicing this technique regularly can change your brain. In one study, people who practiced this technique for eight weeks showed growth in the neural pathways coming in and out of the right prefrontal cortex (Engviv et al. 2012). This part of the brain is responsible for your "mind's eye," where you hold visual information and prep it for encoding and storage.

You can download a worksheet where I guide you through the Roman room method to memorize a list of brain healthy foods at http://newharbinger.com/47438.

Practice Learning Lists: List 3

For list 3, read the following list of words. As you do, categorize and also visualize the items and categories. Draw dramatic pictures (bonus points if you can link them in your drawings by having them interact in some way, such as stacked, grouped, colliding, laid out in a scene, and so forth). After no more than five minutes, write the list items from memory on a sheet of paper.

Ready, go.

- Grass
- Chair
- Stapler
- Lawnmower

- Tree
- Eraser
- Pick
- Table

- Pen
- Rake
- Ruler
- Shovel

- Flower
- Sofa
- Shrub
- Bed

Category 1: _____

Category 2: _____

Category 3: _____

Category 4: _____

Once you've studied your categories and pictures, cover up the material and write the items on a piece of paper.

How many you did you get? Write the total from list 3 here: _____

Learning Lists Exercise Summary

How did your scores pan out?

Total from list 1: _____   Total from list 2: _____   Total from list 3: _____

Did you recall more items as you went along using more strategies?

Elaborate encoding takes effort, but the more you practice these techniques, the more automatic they become. A strong memory doesn't come from a magic pill, it is developed through strategy, effort, and practice, which leads us to the last WOPR strategy: rehearse.

Rehearse

We overestimate the ability of the human memory, assuming we should be able to remember everything perfectly after just one exposure. If you really want your memory to live up to its potential, then you must rehearse what you want to remember. Memory researchers study this by looking at what we call the "learning curve," which is what the graph looks like when we plot the number of items people get on each trial of a memory test. People overwhelmingly tend to get more items on the second and third learning trials of a memory test compared to the first trial. As people get older, they need a couple of more trials to remember the same number of items as younger people (Zimprich, Rast, and Martin 2008). You can utilize this rehearsal skill to your advantage.

Repeat Out Loud

A great way to rehearse new information is to repeat it out loud a couple of times. This is easy to do in a conversation. Simply repeat what the other person said in the form of a question or by paraphrasing. It may seem awkward at first, but you may do it naturally already without realizing it. If it feels foreign to you, I encourage you to practice it because it's also a good social skill. People feel heard and understood, while you remember better.

For example, say you're in New York City and you ask someone to tell you where to find the Empire State Building. They tell you, and you repeat, "The Empire State Building is at the corner of Thirty-Fourth Street and Fifth Avenue, you say?" See, fairly natural.

This is a common tip for remembering the name of someone you just met. The standard recommendation is to try to use the name three times in your first conversation. Repeat the name when you first hear it. "Well, hi Bill Smith. It is great to meet you." Call them by name once during your conversation. "Have you lived here a long time, Bill?" Finally, call them by name again when you end the conversation. "Well, Bill, it was really great meeting you. I hope to see you soon."

It might feel a little weird at first if you don't already do this, but people are usually impressed by this. Don't give up if you forgot the name immediately. It's okay to say, "Please tell me your name again; I'm so sorry." Chances are they've forgotten your name already, too, not because you're not memorable, but because they probably aren't making the effort themselves.

Repeat to Someone Else

You can also rehearse by telling someone else all about it. A teaching method in medical school is "See one, do one, teach one." That last step is an important rehearsal technique that you can use in your everyday life. Recounting an interesting fact you heard on the news, an entertaining story, or a joke is an easy way to rehearse what you want to remember. What will work even better is to rehearse the story to yourself a couple of times, polishing it up before telling someone.

Quiz Yourself

Get into the habit of quizzing yourself. For example, you park your car on the fifth floor of a parking garage. You did a good job of paying attention to the sign indicating what floor you are on, and you took your mental snapshot, but now you need to quiz yourself on the floor number at gradually increasing intervals. Quiz yourself right after looking at the number or right after writing it down, quickly verifying whether you are right or wrong. Getting it right helps because you feel good, giving you a little burst of dopamine, your happy brain chemical, which can improve your memory. Getting it wrong also helps because the disappointment can make what you're trying to remember more salient than if you were to get it right.

Then quiz yourself on your walk to the elevator. If you didn't write the floor number down, you can verify the floor number at the elevator. Quiz yourself again about halfway to your destination and again after you've settled into the event. Quiz yourself again any other time you think about it (for example, when you go to the restroom or when you have a quiet moment to yourself).

Quizzing yourself is also a great study skill. If you've made an outline or study guide for a test, which I hope you have done as part of the organize step in WOPR, then as you look over your study guide, cover the details with your hand or a sheet of paper, only revealing the category or heading, and work to recall the details of the list without looking. Let's practice:

Outline what you've learned about the WOPR step rehearse. (Tip: Look at topic sentences and jot down main ideas.):

- _____

- _____

- _____

- _____

- _____

- _____

- _____

Now study the outline by quizzing yourself, covering up the bullets and only revealing them to check to see whether you're right or wrong.

Now that you're a memory-making machine, growing baby brain cells, giving them jobs, and plumping up your brain, you're ready to move on to some other strategies for brain 401(k) investing. Keep using WOPR and the enhanced strategies you learned in this chapter to help you keep checking items off your brain bucket list, and you can also use them to help you encode all the cool information coming your way in the next chapters.

Chapter 8

Soothe Stress for a Bigger Brain and Greater Focus

You've grown baby brain cells through physical activity and helped them grow up to be new neurons by learning new things. Now we need to turn to improving your focus and helping you keep those brain cells around.

Stress Zaps Memory Now and Later

Stress is an essential part of life. We need it. It keeps us safe, but there are two key ways that it gets in the way of memory. In the short run, stress can zap your concentration and thereby interfere with your memory, and in the long run, chronic stress is hard on your brain, thereby lowering your cognitive reserve. Learning about the neuroscience of stress will help motivate you to better manage your stress, thereby improving your focus and memory and protecting your brain.

Stress affects your memory by stealing important resources from your thinking brain and diverting them to the older parts of your brain that keep you alive. When your survivalistic, fight-flight-freeze response kicks in, which I'll describe in detail below, your attention is understandably drawn toward the things that might kill you. You don't need to be solving math problems while you're running away from a lion. Why does this happen? Well it's all about blood flow.

The human brain makes up only about 2 percent of your total body mass, but it consumes nearly 20 percent of your blood supply at rest (Rink and Khanna 2011). That makes it a very energy-hungry organ. It's so energy hungry that the 20 percent of the blood supply that it is consuming is not even enough to allow the blood flow to be evenly distributed to all parts of the brain at the same time. You do have sort of a low, baseline level of blood flow going to all parts of your brain to keeps brain cells alive, but it's not enough to provide the resources (oxygen and glucose) that neurons need to "fire." When one part of the brain becomes active (when neurons start firing), the cells in that region suck up the lion's share of the blood flow. This is how we measure brain activity. A functional MRI (fMRI) scan, which looks at real-time brain activity, shows where all the newly oxygenated blood is going, and a PET scan measures which parts of the brain are metabolizing the most glucose (or sugar) from the blood (Dale and Halgren 2001).

Two important sections of the human brain are particularly energy hungry, each for entirely different reasons, and knowing this is critically important for your memory. The first section is your prefrontal cortex (PFC), your "thinking brain," which houses memory recall and those important memory-support skills like planning, organizing, and focusing (aka executive functions). The PFC is energy hungry because it is relatively inefficient. Think about how much energy it takes to concentrate and focus; that is your PFC working.

The other energy-hungry region of the brain is your limbic system, or your "emotional brain." It is energy hungry to ensure your survival. When the limbic system gets activated, it sucks most of the blood supply to itself, robbing your PFC of essential blood flow. I know you've experienced what this feels like before, or at least you're probably familiar with the aftereffects. Ever lose an argument? After you walk away and your PFC starts to kick back in, you come up with the *best comeback ever*. You think, *Why didn't I think of that? Okay, I know, I'm gonna text him…*

Your focus is vulnerable to the blood flow draining from your PFC to your limbic system. We call this "limbic hijacking" or an "amygdala hijack" (Goleman 1995). When fear, anger, and even excitement kick in, concentration, and thus memory, can be a real challenge.

What's Your Experience with Limbic Hijacking?

Think back to a situation when you were so consumed by fear, anxiety, excitement, or another emotion that you couldn't think straight. How was your memory affected?

Cindy wrote: The last time my kid came home after curfew, I was so mad. I struggled to make my point and remember examples of her not listening in the past. I couldn't get the words out. I felt like my head was full of bees. I couldn't hear normally. I sort of felt like I was floating, and my chest hurt.

_____

_____

_____

_____

_____

The Long Game: Preserving Your Brain 401(k) and Optimizing Investments

Chronic stress also affects memory in the long run by lowering cognitive reserve and increasing the risk for dementia. The stress hormone cortisol is toxic to brain cells, killing brain cells you've had your whole life and shrinking the hippocampus, (the source of your long-term memory encoding; Burkhardt et al. 2015). This can whittle away at your brain 401(k) over time. Not only that, but cortisol also *inhibits the growth of new brain cells* in and around your hippocampus (Cameron and Gould 1994), making it harder to actively invest in your brain 401(k).

The good news is that you don't have to get rid of all of your stress. In fact, you can't, but you can work to protect your brain from the damaging effects. To optimize your brain 401(k) investing, it is a really good idea to do what health psychologist Kelly McGonigal (2015) recommends, which is to "get better at stress." In this chapter you will learn and practice lots of techniques to get you out of limbic hijacking, help you regain your focus and memory, and protect your memory over time. But first I want you to check in on your stress level.

Stress Self-Assessment

Stress comes in many forms. From trauma to stressful life events, like moving, losing a job, and grieving a death, to daily hassles and the thoughts we think, stress is everywhere. I find it useful to focus on the physical and mental aspects of stress, since that is what we can control. Take a moment to get a sense of how you deal with stress; check all that apply:

- ☐   I worry a lot about the future.
- ☐   I often brood or ruminate about the past.
- ☐   I worry about what people think of me.
- ☐   I get panic attacks.
- ☐   I avoid things that might make me anxious.
- ☐   I hold tension in my face, neck, or shoulders.
- ☐   I hold tension in my chest, torso, back, or stomach.
- ☐   I struggle with digestive issues.
- ☐   My heart often races or pounds for no reason.
- ☐   I am easily startled.
- ☐   I find it hard to sit with my thoughts.
- ☐   I have trouble concentrating.
- ☐   People are often mean to me and hurt my feelings.
- ☐   I sweat a lot.
- ☐   I find myself holding my breath a lot.
- ☐   I have trouble sleeping.
- ☐   I sigh a lot.
- ☐   I never express my fear, hurt, anger, or sadness.
- ☐   I bottle up my feelings until they boil over.
- ☐   I often feel overwhelmed.
- ☐   I get tunnel vision sometimes as if I'm going to pass out.
- ☐   I feel dizzy or floaty when I'm upset or scared.
- ☐   Sometimes I freeze or check out, "lights are on, nobody's home."
- ☐   I have a history of trauma.

The Neuroscience of Stress

A great place to start getting better at stress is to understand the neuroscience of stress. On each side of your brain, you have a tiny almond-shaped structure deep inside your temporal lobe, sitting right in front of your hippocampus, called the amygdala, which you can think of as your "fear detector." It is constantly scanning your environment for things it thinks might kill you. In fact, researchers learned recently that there is a direct fast pathway from the thalamus (what I call Grand Central Station for your brain since all of your sensory information comes to the thalamus first before going elsewhere in the brain) to the amygdala (LeDoux 2012); see figure 8. This means that sensory information gets to your amygdala before it gets to the other, more logical parts of your cortex. Therefore, your amygdala literally knows when there is something that might kill you before you do. This means that your "gut reaction" is real because before you are even aware of what's going on, your amygdala has already decided something is scary and has started mobilizing your body to protect you.

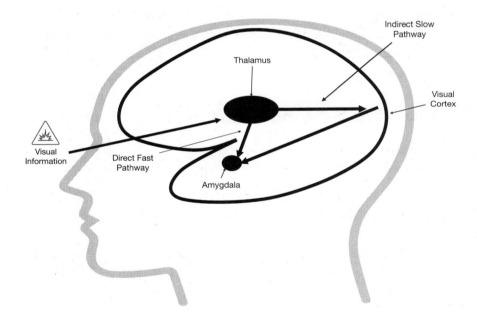

Figure 8. Sensory information travels from the thalamus to the amygdala through the direct fast pathway one hundred times faster than the indirect slow pathway. In this image, the visual danger is received first by the amygdala before it can be processed "consciously" by the visual cortex, which is located on the outer covering of back of the brain and also communicates with the amygdala.

Think back to a time when you reacted automatically to something. Maybe you jumped seeing something out of the corner of your eye, slammed on the breaks in traffic, or screamed when someone touched you. What did you feel in your body? Did you notice any impact on your concentration or memory?

_____

_____

_____

Let's go through that physical reaction. The amygdala triggers the HPA axis, which is a pathway through which hormones are sent from the hypothalamus (H) to the pituitary gland (P) and down to the adrenal glands (A), which are on top of your kidneys, triggering the release of adrenaline into your body. Adrenaline then binds to all of your soft tissues (heart, gut, lungs, muscles, and so forth) to activate your fight-flight-freeze response. _All of this happens automatically, completely outside of your awareness,_ all because your amygdala thought something was going to kill you. Therefore, it's important that you not judge these physical responses, but rather grow to appreciate them.

Your Stress Sensations and What They Mean to You

Think about your heart racing, being short of breath, feeling shaky, feeling dizzy or hot, breaking out in a cold sweat, feeling nauseous, or like you suddenly need to go to the bathroom. What do these sensations mean to you?

Cindy wrote: I hate those feelings. I feel like I'm going to lose control.

_____

_____

How could you reframe that thought into a more helpful thought?

Cindy wrote: Those fight-flight-freeze feelings are helpful. Even though they don't feel good, they let me know when there is something that might hurt me or that makes me mad or scared. I will use this information to protect myself.

_____

_____

_____

_____

Have you ever felt this way when you couldn't remember something or come up with the right word? Journal about a time when this happened recently, and also write what you might be able to do to regain your focus when it happens again.

Cindy wrote: Oh my gosh. I break into a cold sweat every time I can't remember the name of a restaurant or something like that. I think I get scared that I'm getting dementia. I could tell myself that it's okay, and if I relax, then I'll probably remember it later.

_____

_____

_____

_____

(This worksheet is also available for download at http://newharbinger.com/47438.)

You Have More Control Than You Might Think

The early anatomists called the part of your nervous system that controls these automatic body reactions the "autonomic nervous system." It controls the stuff you don't have to think about, like your heart beating, digesting your food, and breathing. Isn't it nice that you don't have to think about breathing to stay alive?

The autonomic nervous system has two divisions: the sympathetic nervous system, which activates the fight-or-flight response, and the parasympathetic nervous system, which does the opposite, what med students call "rest-and-digest." ("Freeze" is not the same as fight-or-flight. It's actually an extreme parasympathetic state, so we aren't going to talk much about it here). Even though the early anatomists called these two divisions separate nervous systems, it's actually more helpful to think of them as two different *states* of the same nervous system because *they cannot both be active at the same time.* You are *either* in fight-or-flight or in rest-and-digest, and this is handy to remember because you actually have more control over your autonomic nervous system than the early anatomists thought when they named it "autonomic." You can control your autonomic nervous system through your breath and muscle tension. If you slow down the breath, you can slow your heart rate and lower your blood pressure; releasing muscle tension triggers this relaxation response as well. Doing this will help you get out of limbic hijack, reengaging your PFC, and help you focus, concentrate, and remember better.

Top-Down Anxiety, aka Worry and Rumination

This automatic, amygdala-based stress is what we call bottom-up stress. The first clue that it's happening may be noticing a change in your body. We humans are unique and special though because we have a second form of stress that we call top-down stress.

In his book *Why Zebras Don't Get Ulcers,* Robert Sapolsky (2004) writes about why zebras don't get ulcers and we do by explaining that most other animal species have a healthy balance between fight-or-flight and rest-and-digest. Zebras are normally just hanging out, eating grass, chilling, until a lion comes along, which triggers a healthy stress response, and the zebras run away. Out of sight, out of mind, they go back to eating grass, digesting their food, flushing out cortisol, and storing up energy for the next time a lion comes along.

We humans, and other social primates, have the unique ability of activating our stress response purely with our thoughts. This is what we call "top-down stress." Because of top-down stress, far too many of us end up in a chronic state of fight-or-flight pumping out too much cortisol, damaging the brain and limiting memory. Unlike zebras, we struggle to "turn it off" and go back to rest-and-digest. Zebras don't obsess about the lion, but we humans do. If you got chased by a lion, how might you react? Could you just go back to eating grass, no big deal? I doubt it. I bet you'd be on the phone calling all of your friends. "You'll never guess what just happened to me. I was almost eaten by a lion." This "analysis" is helpful and adaptive because it allows us to anticipate and plan for terrible future events. However, it can also go haywire, going on too long, reactivating the amygdala over and over, pumping more cortisol into the body and brain, and wreaking havoc on our health.

Interrupting Limbic Hijacking to Reengage Your Focus

Fortunately, there is a lot you can do to interrupt limbic hijacking and restore your nervous system to a healthy balance. What follows is a mix of top-down and bottom-up approaches. I suggest you try them all.

1. Soothe the Amygdala

Soothing the amygdala means that you work to jump into your body to help clear out the fight-or-flight response when it is not serving you. Earlier we talked about the HPA axis, which results in the release of adrenaline and cortisol from the adrenal glands. I didn't mention it before, but one function of cortisol is to travel up to your hypothalamus, signaling the HPA axis to shut itself off rather quickly. The entire process of your amygdala sensing that something might kill you, triggering the HPA axis to release the adrenaline, and then the clearing of all of the chemicals from your body takes less than ninety seconds (Bolte Taylor 2006), *unless the amygdala reactivates the process.* So your body will do what it needs to do to return to homeostasis, but your amygdala needs to be told to cool it sometimes.

Since you can't reason with your amygdala, the best way to soothe it is through the body. Taking a breath will communicate to your amygdala, "Hey, we've got this. It's cool. We're safe. Thank you for trying to save my life. At ease soldier." Breathing will help you loosen yourself from a limbic hijack and reengage your focus so you can remember better.

Soothe the Amygdala with Four-Count Breaths

Take a few moments to practice this very simple breathing exercise. You're simply going to pay attention to your breath while you count to four on the inhale and count to four on the exhale. The trick is to allow the breath to control the rate of counting and not the other way around, so if your breath is short and shallow, you'll count faster than if your breath is slow. Do ten of these, and since your mind will be busy counting, you can keep track of the ten breaths with your fingers. Go ahead...

How was that? Did you notice any changes in your breath or in your body?

_____

_____

_____

_____

2. Meditate

Research on the brain benefits of meditation has been exploding over the past decade or so. Researchers, including Richard Davidson at the University of Wisconsin in Madison, have been doing all sorts of cool experiments looking at the brains of meditators through MRI scanners, including the brain of His Holiness the Dalai Lama himself. Rick Hanson (2009) wrote a book called *Buddha's Brain* in which he summarizes many of the awesome effects of meditation on the brain, including increased overall brain volume (a bigger brain), increased activation and reduced age-related cortical thinning of the prefrontal cortex (the "thinking brain"), and increased gray matter (where the cell bodies live—probably not more cells, but a plumping of the gray matter likely related to more dendrites and connections) in parts of the cortex related to empathy and bonding and in and around the hippocampus (*memory!*).

Meditation also likely rewires the amygdala to make it less jumpy and a source of distraction. People who are more mindful have smaller amygdalae (Taren, Creswell, and Gianaros 2013), while people with chronic stress, anxiety, and clinical depression have bigger amygdalae (Andrade and Kumar Rao 2010). As of the writing of this book, no study has shown that you can shrink your amygdala by meditating, but I'm willing to bet real money that that study is coming.

High-Definition Memories

The way I think about the relationship between mindfulness meditation practice and memory reminds me of the time about fifteen years ago when my husband bought his first high-definition TV. We were young; I was still in graduate school. He got a second job and saved up his money to buy a big, fancy plasma TV. He was so excited. He got it up on the wall, plugged it in, and the picture was *terrible*. We both thought, *What the…?* So he called the satellite company and told them his problem. They quickly informed him, "Oh yeah. You're running the regular-definition signal into the TV. You have to pay an extra five dollars a month to get a high-definition signal." This was about the same time when I was learning about mindfulness, and I thought to myself, *That's what mindfulness does for memory. It helps you have "high-definition" memories.* When you practice mindfulness, you take in more of the present moment, more details. The bandwidth is higher, so the memories are richer.

Mindfulness meditation is nothing new. It has existed for centuries in Eastern cultures, evolving into Buddhist practices and yoga traditions. Jon Kabat-Zinn and many others have "Westernized" these old Eastern traditions and helped develop them into therapeutic interventions, such as mindfulness-based stress reduction (MBSR). Dr. Kabat-Zinn defines mindful meditation as "paying attention in a particular way: on purpose, in the present moment, and nonjudgmentally" (Kabat-Zinn 1994, 4). See that? *Paying attention.* Research studies have shown that even a very low dose of meditation practice (four twenty-minute sessions) can improve working memory and other executive function skills (Zeidan et al. 2010). The more you are aware of the present moment, the more you can remember. Meditation also functions as one of the best forms of attention training available today (Mitchell, Zylowska, and Kollins 2015).

Let's break down Dr. Kabat-Zinn's definition of mindfulness as we prepare to practice this technique.

1. *Pay attention.* This is simple enough and right on target.

2. *On purpose.* Be intentional; this is something you are deciding to do.

3. *In the present moment.* This is where the "memory making" happens.

4. *Nonjudgmentally.* Don't get mad at yourself when your mind wanders, because it will. Kindly redirect yourself back to the present moment and reengage—that's how focus works.

One Minute of Present-Moment Awareness

Set a timer for one minute. If one minute feels overwhelming, start with fifteen or thirty seconds, but I challenge you to one full minute. Pay attention to the present moment, nonjudgmentally; keep redirecting your focus back to the present moment and see how it goes.

How did it go? What did you notice? What did you do when your mind wandered?

_____

_____

_____

_____

Set Some Meditation Goals

First, flip back to chapter 2 to reference the attention goals you identified there. How have you been keeping up with these? What would you like to tweak in your plan? If you want to be more intentional about your goal, what systems will you put into place to help you with that? Take a moment to journal about your attention plan moving forward.

_____

_____

_____

_____

_____

What meditation approach do you want to practice (for example, four-count breath, present-moment awareness, guided audio, and so forth)?

_____

_____

Goal. How often will you practice this and for how long each time?

_____

_____

Reward. How will you reward yourself for accomplishing your goal? You may need to bribe yourself to do it (for example, giving yourself a squirt of perfume or watching a TV show).

_____

3. Work the Worry Plan

Worry and rumination, those "top-down" sources of anxiety, are known to lead to anxiety and depression, which are known risk factors for dementia in the long run and zap your memory in the short run by distracting you from the present moment. "Worry thoughts," which often include the phrase "What if...," tend to be about the future and are associated with feelings of anxiety. "Rumination thoughts," which are often of the "should of, could of, would of" variety, tend to be about the past and are associated with depressed feelings. So you can see how these mind states can really detract from your memory. As the famous Harvard psychology professor Ellen Langer says when people are not there, "they're not there to know that they're not there" (Langer 2014).

A downside of brain plasticity (cells that wire together fire together) is that the more you worry and ruminate, the more likely you are to worry and ruminate. The more you worry and ruminate, the more you activate your amygdala, triggering your fight-or-flight response, hijacking your concentration and memory, and the more sensitive your amygdala becomes, making it jumpier and more likely to be activated (Hanson 2009). So what should you do? Well I've got a plan, but first let's capture some of those worry thoughts.

Worry Exercise

What do you worry about? List those thoughts here (skip the right-hand column for now, we will come back to it). You know something is a worry thought when it starts with "What if..."

Worry (Write your worry thoughts here.)	Plan (Make a plan.)

Worry serves a purpose in that it helps us plan. The way to deal with worry is to use it as nature intended, by planning for how to deal with that terrible thing you imagine. It doesn't have to be a twelve-point comprehensive disaster plan. In their book *Rewire Your Anxious Brain*, Catherine Pittman and Elizabeth Karle (2015) wrote about the worry plan, which has three steps: (1) worry, (2) plan, (3) stop. Once you have your plan, the worry thought is no longer useful because you've already put it to good use by making the plan. You don't need to think about that problem anymore. It is solved for now. The thing is not happening right now, so don't rob the potential joy of this moment (and awareness, focus, and memories of this moment) by worrying and borrowing trouble. Worry, plan, stop.

Go back up to your list above, and insert a plan for each of the items on your list. Here are some examples from our friend Cindy:

Worry	Plan
What if I'm getting dementia?	Then I will find some help.
What if my son gets in a car accident?	It will be tough, but I will get through it.
What if my house burns down?	I have insurance, and I'll scan my photos.

I hope that you now understand the role that fear and anxiety play in interrupting your memory. This is a very important area that most of us need to focus on. It is especially critical for those with memory changes and those who have been told that their memory is fine but who are still worried. Limbic hijacking is one of the biggest sources of memory disruption, so becoming skilled at getting your focus back "online" will do wonders for your daily memory function.

Chapter 9

Sleep

In high-powered corporate and medical circles, sleep has been historically undervalued. People often brag about how little sleep they need, but science doesn't support this way of thinking. Fortunately, sleep is having a renaissance. When it comes to your memory, now and in the future, getting plenty of sleep is essential.

Sleep Helps Your Memory Now

Sleep is critical to helping you have a sharp memory. Lack of sleep leads to sharp declines in attention and executive function. The dulling of reaction time from a poor night's sleep is on par with being drunk (Williamson and Feyer 2000). As I have mentioned several times in this book, attention is the gateway to memory. A good memory requires sharp focus. You can't expect yourself to remember things that you never noticed in the first place, right? A dulled attention is the first way that lack of sleep impairs memory.

The rapid eye movement (REM) stage of sleep is necessary for retaining new long-term memories. During REM, your hippocampus is very active, consolidating your long-term memories into "really long-term memories" that you will hold on to (Siegel 2001). Ever notice the effect of "sleeping on it" when learning something or studying for a test? Suddenly the next morning you know the material a whole lot better because it was "consolidated" during your REM sleep.

Sleep Quantity Matters

Sleeping a full seven to eight hours is the goal for practically everyone. There is probably a margin of error, but you really do need a full night of sleep each night, or most nights. Sleeping too little (fewer than six hours per night) and sleeping too much (nine or more hours) increases the risk for stroke. Seven hours per night is ideal in terms of stroke risk, and the further you move away from this number in either direction, the more your risk increases (Phua, Jayaram, and Wijeratne 2017).

A big reason for this has to do with getting enough REM sleep, because most of your REM sleep occurs during the second half of the night. The first half of the night is mostly deep sleep, which is also important, as I will describe below, but to get all of the REM your memory needs, you need to

sleep past that fifth, sixth, and maybe even seventh hour (McCarley 2007). REM sleep is also important for calming the amygdala, your fear detector (Van der Helm et al. 2011). When people don't get
enough REM sleep, the amygdala is significantly more reactive, and as you've been learning, amygdala and limbic hijacking can get in the way of your memory by distracting you and stealing your
focus.

Here's the thing about getting in all of those REM cycles. You must stay asleep throughout the
night. If you're awake longer than thirty minutes, your sleep cycles start over, which means you probably won't have time to get in all those REM cycles. Isn't that a bummer?

If you snore, please go see your doctor. Sleep apnea is a serious health risk, increasing the risk for
heart attack and stroke, and it diminishes your attention and executive function (those higher-level
thinking skills that a good memory relies on; Moyer et al. 2001).

The issue with sleep apnea is that your airway may collapse when your muscles relax during sleep.
Your brain works hard to keep you alive, and if it detects that you're not getting the air you need, then
it will wake you up. The frequent waking is what tends to affect concentration and memory. So talk
to your doctor. There are lots of sleep apnea treatments with new and better ones emerging all the
time, so even if you've tried something it the past and hated it, try again.

Let's digest. Jot down your reactions to all of this information. Are you surprised? Do you have questions?
Any ideas for adjusting your sleep?

What Is Keeping You Up at Night?

☐ Worry

☐ TV

☐ Too many trips to the bathroom

☐ My snoring

☐ My bed-partner's snoring

☐ Restless legs

☐ Too many thoughts

☐ Too much coffee

☐ Medication side effects

☐ Not tired at night, but tired in the day

☐ Napping all day

☐ Kids

☐ Baby

☐ Night sweats

☐ Nightmares

☐ _____

☐ _____

☐ _____

The Impact of Sleep on Memory in the Long Run

Sleep was not a top brain 401(k) investing strategy until relatively recently. The most exciting thing about recent sleep discoveries is that sleep may be the first real, direct preventer of actual Alzheimer's pathology. All the other factors we have been targeting for brain 401(k) investing so far deal with building up your cognitive reserve so you have more brain cells available. With more brain cells, your brain can better withstand damage. Sleep builds up the cognitive reserve, too, but it may also prevent the actual accumulation of those beta-amyloid plaques that cause Alzheimer's disease.

Deep sleep, the cycles you have early in the night, seem to represent the lymphatic system of the brain, where toxins get flushed out. The body has lymph nodes that carry toxins out of the body. Until recently, we didn't know if the brain had a detox system like this, but it does, which is cleverly called the "glymphatic system" (Jessen et al. 2015).

During deep sleep, the glial cells in the brain shrink by 20 percent, allowing the spinal fluid in your brain to flush out toxins (De Vivo et al. 2017). (Glial cells are the "other" cells in your brain that aren't neurons but are important for holding neurons in place, metabolizing nutrients, and "cleaning up" toxins.) The beta-amyloid plaques that cause Alzheimer's disease are one of the toxins that gets flushed out. Getting plenty of deep sleep, therefore, may help you flush these plaques out of your brain before they can damage your cells (Jessen et al. 2015). Not getting enough sleep, though, may make the beta-amyloid plaques stick in your brain, leading to Alzheimer's disease.

Recent research is challenging the old assumption that people need less sleep as they get older. It's common for people to sleep fewer hours per night as they age, which we just assumed was normal. However, Matthew Walker and his colleagues at the University of California at Berkley recently discovered that adults who sleep fewer hours in their fifties, sixties, and seventies have more beta-amyloid plaques stuck in their brains (Winer et al. 2019). Now this is a simple correlation, so we can't draw any conclusions on which causes which. Beta-amyloid may cause people to stay awake, or sleeping less causes the plaque to stick in the brain. Without better studies, we don't know yet. Since we can't bust up amyloid in the brain yet (at least not as of the writing of this book), we can work to help older adults sleep longer and see if that has an impact on preventing Alzheimer's.

Let's process. What are your thoughts right now about sleep? Are you worried, inspired, confused? Take some time to jot down your thoughts and reactions.

_____

_____

_____

_____

_____

There is a lot you can do to improve your sleep. You may even know what to do, but, like a lot of people, you may struggle to stay motived. Now that you know the impact sleep has on your memory, you may be a bit more motivated to improve your sleep patterns. I've listed sleep recommendations below, but first let's talk a little about meds.

Sleep Medications Can Affect Memory Formation

It's common to wish for a pill to take care of all of this, right? I get it. However, most sleep medications negatively affect memory in one way or another.

Prescription Sleep Medications

The class of drugs called benzodiazepines (which includes Xanax and Klonopin) are known to block memory formation (Savić et al. 2005) and interfere with neuroplasticity in the hippocampus (Del Cerro, Jung, and Lynch 1992), the activity you need to form new memories. Benzos are also highly addictive. Unless you're taking them to control something like sleepwalking, then I suggest talking to your doctor about alternatives.

I Sure Love My Tylenol PM

You might think over-the-counter (OTC) sleep medications are safer and better for your memory than prescription drugs, but buyer beware. There is mounting concern about the impact OTC sleep aids have on memory and the risk for dementia. Here's why.

All OTC sleep aids are antihistamines. All antihistamines are anticholinergic, meaning they lower the amount of acetylcholine in your brain (Church and Church 2013). Acetylcholine is your memory neurotransmitter, the juice your hippocampus uses to form new memories. Therefore, antihistamines do the opposite of what memory-boosting drugs (which increase acetylcholine transmission), like Aricept, do.

We know that anticholinergic drugs, like antihistamines, increase the risk of dementia in people who already have mild cognitive changes, particularly women. Therefore, getting women with mild memory declines off these medications is a top priority for preventing dementia (Artero et al. 2008). I encourage everyone to reconsider using antihistamines for sleep given both the immediate impact on memory and the potential long-term risk.

If you have allergies, don't fret. Not all antihistamines enter your brain, only those that make you sleepy. There is little memory risk with "nondrowsy" antihistamines, like Claritin or Zyrtec.

As of the writing of this book, melatonin seems to be the safest solution for sleep, at least in terms of your memory now and later on. Some shorter-acting prescription sleep medications may also be safe and effective for your insomnia. However, every sleep medication or supplement has potential side effects and may disrupt your sleep cycles. The bottom line is to discuss all of this with your doctor and to consider nonmedication interventions for improving your sleep.

What questions do you have for your doctor about sleep medications?

_____

_____

_____

_____

_____

Nonmedication Strategies for Better Sleep

The safest approach to improving sleep is through nonmedical means, so here are some lifestyle strategies for improving your sleep in order to boost your memory.

1. Pay Attention to Stimulants

If you're on a stimulant medication, like Ritalin or Provigil, talk to your doctor about optimal dosing and timing to optimize your sleep. Set yourself a caffeine curfew and consider limiting desserts before bed. Nicotine, alcohol, and sugar can also function as stimulants, potentially making it harder to fall asleep or stay asleep.

What is your stimulant plan?

_____

_____

_____

_____

_____

_____

2. Keep a Regular Bedtime and Wake Time

Your body thrives on rhythm. Your brain is pumping out hormones, like melatonin at night to help you drift to sleep, and cortisol in the morning to wake you up, all to help you maintain that rhythm. So help your brain out a little will ya?

Your bedtime: _____ Your wake time: _____

Be sure to put alerts in your smartphone, if you have one; set alarms elsewhere in your home for both your bedtime and wake times.

3. Have a Wind-Down Routine

Speaking of melatonin, you can help your body produce more melatonin by giving yourself a wind-down routine. It doesn't have to be superelaborate, maybe just a few rules and routines that you set for yourself, like having a screen curfew, brushing your teeth, washing your face, turning on some "spa music" or a guided meditation.

Your wind-down routine start time: _____

Your wind-down routine includes:

_____   _____

_____   _____

_____   _____

4. Be More Active During the Day

Physical activity releases muscle tension, and the endorphins your brain releases with activity could last up to four days. Just be careful not to be active too close to bedtime since it can also be energizing.

How is your physical activity routine going so far? What if anything can you do to stay motivated, kick it up a notch, or make an improvement?

_____

_____

_____

_____

_____

5. Keep Nighttime Wake-Up Times Short

Knowing sleep cycles start over after being awake for longer than thirty minutes means that you'll likely want to work much harder to keep any wake-ups you have during the night as short as possible. A quick pee, sip of water, and back to bed. I'm the type of person whose thoughts don't stop, so I like to turn on an audio recording that is hypnotic in some way. Meditation tracks are great for this, but be sure to pick tracks that don't require a lot of focus and will lull you back to sleep.

What's your middle-of-the-night plan?

_____

_____

_____

_____

Let's Get Ahold of Those Thoughts

If you are like me and the numerous thoughts running through your head are a big barrier to sleeping, you can use the next exercise to get ahold of them and maybe do something about them. Getting your thoughts on paper is really helpful. For one, the reason the thought may be on a loop inside your mind is your brain's attempt to help you remember it for when you need it later. If you write it down, voila, it's securely rememberable outside your mind. *(The following thought-log worksheet is also available at http://newharbinger.com/47438.)*

Midnight Thought Log

Step 1. Leave your workbook on your nightstand tonight with a pen inserted at this page, and if you wake up in the middle of the night with a string of thoughts running through your head, write them here.

_____

_____

_____

_____

_____

_____

_____

_____

_____

_____

Step 2. Ask yourself a couple of questions to help soothe yourself, like *What's so terrible about that? Could I handle it? What would I tell my friend if she came to me with that issue?* Also, don't forget the worry plan from chapter 8. Worry is functional in that it helps us plan. See if you can quickly come up with a plan. Write it or any other supportive thoughts below.

_____

_____

_____

_____

_____

_____

_____

_____

_____

_____

Now do a body scan and go back to sleep.

Body Scan

Another way to trigger the relaxation response in your brain is by releasing muscle tension in your body. A body scan is a simple and effective way to do that. We have the ability to relax our muscles with our thoughts. Start at the tip-top of your head and scan down your body. You can imagine that your body is full of cortisol (that stress hormone that is toxic to brain cells if it's not flushed out on a regular basis), and as you scan down your body, imagine the cortisol is draining out of you, like water draining out of a bathtub. As the cortisol drains from each part of your body, imagine that part is completely relaxed, passing over your forehead, eyebrows, eye sockets, cheeks, jaw, lips, tongue, chin, base of the skull, neck, shoulders, upper arms, elbows, forearms, wrists, hands, fingers, chest, upper back and shoulder blades, middle back, abdomen, low back, hips, seat, thighs, knees, shins and calves, ankles, feet, and down into the toes, and out through the drain. Spend a couple of moments, maybe three to five breath cycles here, just enjoying this feeling of total relaxation throughout your body.

How was that? What did you notice in your body?

_____

_____

I hope that sleep now is a bigger priority for you, and when you're struggling to sleep, you have some new tools to make it happen. Many of the skills in this book work together; for example, moving more can help you sleep better. Let's keep exploring more skills as you continue to build your brain and memory.

Chapter 10

Eat Your Veggies

Volumes have been written on diet and the brain. There is a lot we know, and there is still a lot we don't know. I don't agree yet that everyone needs to give up gluten, except for obviously those diagnosed with celiac disease or a similar condition. That said, there are a lot of "memory culprits" in our food supply. The food you put into your body matters quite a lot when it comes to your overall long-term brain health. The short-term effects of food on memory can be a bit more subtle, but I bet if you start experimenting with this, you may find foods that do rob you of your focus by making you feel sluggish or spaced-out, and other foods that help you feel sharper.

How Does Diet Matter?

The field of brain health was first turned on to the importance of diet by epidemiological studies that found that people living in the Mediterranean regions of Italy and Greece had really low rates of Alzheimer's disease. After controlling for every variable they could think of, the researchers concluded that the diet made the difference (Trichopoulou et al. 2003). Since then, several experimental and longitudinal studies have shown that the Mediterranean diet and other similar diets like the MIND diet (Morris et al. 2015) and the MAD diet (a modified Atkins diet; Brandt et al. 2019) help slow cognitive decline, lower the risk of dementia, and in some cases even boost cognition (Martínez-Lapiscina et al. 2013; Brandt et al. 2019).

Diet matters to your brain and memory by the impact it has on (1) your cardiovascular system, (2) blood sugar spikes, and (3) the nutrients your brain needs for optimal memory performance.

Heart and Vascular Health

We've known for a long time that what's good for your heart is good for your brain. Brain cells require constant blood flow to stay alive because they can't store their own energy. To survive and function, they rely on fresh oxygen and glucose (sugar) from the blood. Any interruption in blood flow to the brain, even for a couple of minutes, can lead to massive cell death. Therefore, it is vital that you protect your heart and vasculature to protect your brain and memory. A heart attack stops the supply of freshly oxygenated blood to your brain, and having clogged arteries will cause a stroke or otherwise deprive your brain of adequate blood flow.

We know that diets high in saturated fats, carbohydrates, sodium, and nitrates can damage your cardiovascular system, so this holds true for your brain as well. A heart-healthy diet is a brain-healthy diet. The DASH diet, a diet for lowering blood pressure, was shown to lower dementia risk (Sacks et al. 1999), and diets like the Mediterranean and MIND diets are also generally "heart healthy" as well. There is not a lot of red meat in these diets, fats tend to be polyunsaturated, and there tends to be a plethora of fish and fresh fruits and veggies. People in the Mediterranean region don't seem to eat a lot of french fries, steak, sausage, or chicken nuggets. Olive oil is the primary oil used for dressings and cooking, which is an unsaturated fat, meaning it doesn't solidify inside your arteries the way butter or animal fat does, leading to less buildup of plaque, which can lead to heart attacks and strokes.

Let's digest. *(Get it?)* How are you feeling about what you are learning? Are you seeing any ideas yet for ways you might change your diet to maximize your memory or lower your risk for dementia?

_____

_____

_____

Blood Sugar Spikes

When your blood sugar gets super high, your red blood cells can swell and block blood flow into the tips of your capillaries (small blood vessels at the ends of your arteries—many of these capillaries extend into the middle of your brain). You've probably heard of diabetic neuropathy, when people lose feeling in their fingers or toes or have kidney damage (nephropathy) or damage to their retinas (retinopathy). What all these parts of the body (fingertips, toes, kidneys, eyeballs, middle of your brain) have in common is that they are fed by heavy capillary beds. If a person is losing feeling in their fingers or toes, you can bet that similar damage is happening deep inside their brain.

This matters to memory because the nerve pathways coming in and out of your frontal lobes are fed by these capillaries and these pathways are essential for memory recall, pulling memories out of your mind. These nerve pathways are also vulnerable to small vascular damage from clogged arteries or spikes in blood pressure. Over time, poor vascular health or diabetes can result in an accumulation of damage that results in what we traditionally call "vascular dementia," or what is now called "vascular neurocognitive disorder." Diabetes can also damage your blood vessels, given that this red-blood-cell swelling damages the arterial walls, leading to plaque and scarring.

There are lots of reasons beyond diet why people develop hypertension, arterial plaque, and diabetes, particularly genetic reasons. I don't want this info to sound blaming or shaming. Diet is one part of the bigger picture, but I'm mentioning it here because I find that many people either do not fully understand or appreciate the association between these vascular risk factors and memory. Diet does affect vascular health and diabetes, so it is important to consider the impact of diet on memory via these important risk-factor channels.

Even if you don't have diabetes, this red-blood-cell swelling could happen with a fully functioning pancreas (the organ that produces insulin to regulate your blood sugar). Bingeing on ice cream or Oreos could spike your blood sugar enough to at least disrupt your overall brain chemistry and thereby your concentration, and we know that a low-glycemic diet (a diet low in sugar and carbs designed to keep the blood sugar stable by avoiding blood sugar spikes and dips) seems to be ideal for long-term brain health.

The Mediterranean and MIND diets are low-glycemic. Honey, dates, and fresh fruits make up the bulk of the sweets in these diets. Compare that to donuts and pecan pie. There also isn't a ton of refined pasta or mashed potatoes. The grains are typically in their whole form, like whole-grain rice and whole-grain bread. This means that blood sugar spikes are less common.

It is worth noting that as of the writing of this book, the ketogenic (modified Atkins, or MAD) diet is gaining some new attention. This diet also aims to keep blood sugar levels low. One preliminary study out of Johns Hopkins has shown some early positive results in terms of improving memory (Brandt et al. 2019). A couple of things to note though are that this was a very small study, and the science is very young. Also, ketogenic diets can be hard to stick with and may cause kidney damage, so please proceed with caution and talk with your doctor.

Let's digest. *(This still cracks me up.)* How are you feeling about all of this blood sugar stuff? Are you seeing any ideas yet for ways you might change your diet to maximize your memory or lower your risk for dementia?

_____

_____

_____

Nutrients Needed for Optimal Memory Performance

A couple of nutrients seem key for brain health: omega-3s and antioxidants. Omega-3 fatty acids—found in seafood, nuts, seeds (like chia seeds, flaxseeds, and walnuts), and plant oils (such as flaxseed oil, soybean oil, and canola oil)—keep cell membranes healthy, particularly in the brain and the heart. Participants in the Rush Memory and Aging Project, one of the biggest longitudinal (tracking people over time) studies on lifestyle and dementia to date, who ate seafood at least once a week did better on tests of memory and other thinking skills over the five years they were tracked than participants who didn't eat seafood (Van de Rest et al. 2016). Fish oil supplements seem to be less effective. Fish can be high in mercury, a neurotoxin itself, so don't overdo it. But do eat fish because it seems that the risk of not eating fish at all is worse than the risk of mercury negatively affecting your brain (Morris et al. 2016).

Antioxidants are also critical for long-term brain health. They are helpful to all of your cells because they prevent oxidative stress. I thought for a long time that oxidative stress was something people at health food stores made up to sell vitamins, but it turns out it's a real thing. Oxidative stress describes the burden placed on the body by unstable molecules called "free oxygen radicals" or "free radicals." When oxygen is metabolized (a process called oxidation), some of the oxygen molecules end up missing an electron, making them unstable, so they become free radicals. In their search for that electron to make them stable, these free radicals bounce all around damaging your cells. Oxidation is the same process that causes metal to rust, so you can think of oxidative stress as your body rusting—eek! Antioxidants provide the missing electron these oxygen cells need to stabilize, so antioxidants tone down the oxidative stress in your body and in your brain, allowing more brain cells to stick around in your cognitive reserve.

Antioxidants are simply vitamins and minerals that you already know are good for you. They include vitamins C and E, beta-carotene, and the minerals zinc and selenium. Flavonoids are a particular type of antioxidant that give fruits and veggies their color. They are in pretty much all fruits, vegetables, and herbs, as well as beans, whole grains, red wine, green and black teas, and cocoa. "Superfoods" that are especially high in antioxidants include wild blueberries, red beans, cranberries, and artichoke hearts. Many of the antioxidants are found in the skins of fruits and vegetables, including potatoes and apples—so peeling or boiling these foods may reduce the amount of antioxidants in them. Dark chocolate is one of those "miracle foods" that is also high in antioxidants. But be careful. In order to make it taste so good, it is mixed with a lot of sugar and fat.

Antioxidants are thought to play a role in brain plasticity and long-term potentiation, that process we talked about earlier by which cells wire together. Some experiments have shown enhanced memory performance after ingesting flavonoids (Socci et al. 2017).

Our bodies are better at absorbing the nutrients directly from foods than from supplements, so it's best to try to get antioxidants and omega-3s from your diet. Plus, if you're busy eating lots of fruits and veggies, there is less room in your tummy for the stuff that may block your arteries or cause your red blood cells to swell up.

Let's digest. (One more time!) How are you feeling about all of this omega-3 and antioxidant stuff? Any ideas for changes to your diet?

_____

_____

_____

Your Weekly Brain Diet Checklist

Most of these studies on diet and memory were conducted by having people fill out food-frequency questionnaires. The studies analyze how often people ate foods deemed to be brain healthy versus foods determined to be "potentially harmful." Foods aren't inherently "bad"; it's more about how often you eat them. You're doing a fantastic job if you can check the boxes below:

Did your week look like this?	✓
Used mostly olive oil instead of butter.	
Had at least one green leafy veggie per day on average (green lettuce, kale, greens, spinach, and so forth.	
Had at least one other veggie per day.	
Ate berries at least twice this week.	
Ate nuts on most days.	
Had less than 1 tablespoon of butter or margarine per day.	
Didn't have any cheese this week.	
Ate whole grains at least three times.	
Had fish (not fried) at least once.	
Ate beans three times.	
Ate poultry (not fried) at least twice.	
Ate red meat no more than three times.	
Ate sweets no more than four times.	

(You can download a printable copy of this checklist at http://newharbinger.com/47438.)

Your Brain Diet Plan

Most often eating better is less about knowing what to do and really more about getting ourselves to actually do it, right? Volumes have been written on tricks and methods to improve our diets. Generally, having a plan and some social support is what leads to the best results. So I'd like to help you do that.

The trick about the plan is to make it doable. Often, we don't follow through on goals because we make them too hard or too complicated. If you feel any sort of resistance to any of the goals you identify, it's important to cut that goal in half, and then if you still feel resistance, cut it in half again, and again, and again, until it seems like a doable step. Also, your plan may be more about adding in certain foods instead of taking away certain foods, because if you're eating more fish, beans, fresh fruits, and veggies, then there is less room in your belly for other things like chips and cake.

This is not the time to beat yourself up. It seems that lots of people ebb and flow in their eating patterns. You might be rocking a brain healthy diet already. You might be learning this stuff for the first time. You may want to make subtle changes. You may want to make big changes. Ultimately, it really is up to you because you are in charge.

So What's Your Plan?

You may want to start by adding more fish and fresh veggies to your meals, or you may want to go "all in" by meeting with a nutritionist or joining a diet plan.

Cindy wrote: Gotta cut back on the wine and switch to red for flavonoids. I'll measure it and leave the bottle in the kitchen, Mondays will be fish night (meatless Mondays). I'll stock up on beans, berries, and veggies and only buy one bag of chips for the kids per week.

What is your plan?

_____

_____

_____

_____

_____

_____

Foods you want to eat more of:

_____   _____

_____   _____

_____   _____

_____   _____

Foods you want to eat less of:

_____   _____

_____   _____

_____   _____

_____   _____

People who are going to support you in your new eating habits:

Person	When and How You Will Ask for Their Help

Like I said at the beginning of the chapter, there is a lot we could discuss related to diet and memory. I invariably left things out, like the impact of pesticides and the benefits of organic foods. My overall goal is to give you some basics that you can start with to improve your memory by what you put in your body. Happy chomping!

Chapter 11

Mind Your Meds

So many pills and substances affect memory that I can't possibly address them all. My aim with this chapter is to arm you with enough information to empower you to talk with your doctor about the memory pros and cons of your medications. There is no magic pill to fix your memory. I hope that's clear by now, but there may be some things you and your doctor can do to tune up your memory by addressing your medications, supplements, and other substances.

Medications That Boost Memory

Let's start with the good stuff. There are medications to boost memory. A group of medicines called "cholinesterase inhibitors" include the drugs Aricept (donepezil) and Exelon (rivastigmine). They improve the function of the hippocampus (the structure that stores your long-term memories) by boosting the amount of acetylcholine (your memory neurotransmitter and the juice the hippocampus uses to operate) in the brain. They are only given to people with Alzheimer's disease and a handful of other progressive dementias, like Lewy body dementia, once the memory decline is significant. Another drug called Namenda (memantine) boosts memory for people in the middle to late stages of dementia (Livingston et al. 2017).

These drugs are not given to people without documented memory problems, and current recommendations encourage doctors to not even give them to people with mild neurocognitive disorder (also called mild cognitive impairment or MCI). This is because less than 40 percent of people with MCI go on to develop dementia within three to ten years (Mitchell and Shiri-Feshki 2009).

Memory Supplements

Be skeptical of any supplement touting memory enhancement, and there are a lot. It's easy to get swept up in the claims made by these supplement distributors. The bottom line when it comes to memory supplements is that pretty much every single supplement that has been touted for improving memory, things like Prevagen and gingko biloba, either have not been tested at all, have not been tested in humans, or when tested in humans have not consistently performed better than a placebo. Supplement manufacturers do not have to prove their claims, and active ingredient levels can vary widely from brand to brand and batch to batch. My concern when it comes to supplements is that most are not worth the money. Even omega-3 and antioxidant supplements seem to have limited effectiveness in terms of long-term brain health (Van de Rest et al. 2016); you are way better off getting these nutrients from your food. You may need to buy supplements if you have a specific deficiency, like B_{12}, diagnosed by your doctor, but otherwise I'd prefer you spend your money on things that will help you more, like a personal trainer.

Attention Meds

Don't forget that you can't remember what you don't notice, so a solid attention is also critical for a good memory. Stimulants, like caffeine, can provide a boost in attention for most people, which is probably a big reason why Starbucks is so profitable. Most ADHD medications, like Ritalin and Adderall, are stimulants, as well as other drugs like Provigil. Doctors work to limit their use when they can because of the high potential for abuse. They are similar in many ways to illegal drugs like cocaine and methamphetamine. Under the right circumstance though, stimulant medications can be used, under a doctor's care, to improve focus and memory.

I'd say that unless you've had a brain injury, stroke, or really seemed to have had ADHD as a kid (ADHD is a childhood disorder; there is no such thing as adult-onset ADHD), which persisted into adulthood, then you probably don't need a stimulant medication. Your goals for improved attention and memory are likely best met through meditation, sleep, emotion regulation, and behavior change.

Medications That Get in the Way

There are lots of medications that can limit memory, including many psychiatric medications, such as benzodiazepines (for example Xanax and Klonopin), antipsychotics, older antidepressants, anti-epilepsy drugs, sleep medications, heart drugs (such as beta-blockers), opiates, and marijuana. Some of these drugs block memory formation directly, and others impair memory by way of making you less alert.

Some medications affect memory because they are anticholinergic, meaning they impede your memory neurotransmitter acetylcholine. Thus, these medications work in the opposite way to Aricept by reducing acetylcholine in the brain. As we discussed in the sleep chapter, anticholinergic medications also increase the risk for dementia in older women who already have some mild memory decline (Livingston at al. 2017). Anticholinergic medications include all sedating antihistamines—every over-the-counter sleep aid (except melatonin)—as well as some bladder and psychiatric medications (for example, Seroquel is a powerful antihistamine).

If you are taking any of these medications, it is important that you discuss with your doctor any potential memory side effects and work together on a cost-benefit analysis of your medications.

Keep a List of Your Meds on You

If you take any medication or supplement (prescribed or over the counter), it's a good idea to keep a list on you in case of emergency or for when talking to your doctor. Make a list of your meds—write it down or print it out—and put it in your wallet or wherever makes sense so you always have it with you.

Delirium

As you get older, it is critical that you work closely with your doctor to ensure that your mix of medications and their doses are optimal for your memory. The doses of medications that are processed by the liver are based on estimates of how much of the medication will be cleared by your liver enzymes before getting to your brain. The liver of a seventy-year-old person produces far fewer enzymes than a thirty-year-old person, so doses need to be adjusted accordingly, otherwise too much medication may enter the brain. Medication toxicity is a common cause of "delirium," a temporary disruption in memory usually due to a chemical imbalance. In older adults delirium is often the result of liver changes.

Summarize Your Questions for You Doctor

What are your questions for your doctor about memory meds, supplements, attention meds, the potential memory side effects of medications, and doses and combinations? (Flip back to chapter 9 where you wrote down sleep medication questions to make sure you include those here too.)

_____

_____

_____

_____

_____

_____

_____

Tying One On with My Buddies

Let's face it, sometimes we are not all that kind to our brains. Overdoing it with alcohol can certainly make you foggy and less productive. Mild drinking seems fine for your brain, and there is even some evidence that mild drinkers are less likely to get dementia than teetotalers (Sabia et al. 2018). We aren't really sure why exactly, and I'm certainly not suggesting that you start drinking if you don't already. Not drinking has its own advantages of providing mental clarity. Ultimately, it's a personal choice you make based on how you feel when you use alcohol, including how you sleep at night and how you feel the next day. If you've had some brain damage though, your tolerance for alcohol may be significantly lowered, and the cognitive-altering effects could be much more pronounced.

It's important to be clear and honest with yourself about what "mild-to moderate drinking" really is. We humans are fabulous at rationalizing our behaviors, so what is mild to some may be more like heavy drinking in medical terms. The latest data shows that drinking more than fourteen drinks per week increases your risk for dementia (Sabia et al. 2018). Keep in mind that a standard drink is one and a half ounces of hard liquor, like whisky or vodka (40 percent alcohol by volume, ABV); five ounces of wine (15 percent ABV); or twelve ounces of beer (5 percent ABV).

Let's Get Real About Your Drinking

Think back over the past week and be honest. How many drinks have you had in the last seven days?

_____ Is it above fourteen?

Now divide that number by seven. What is your average number of drinks per day? _____

That is what we call a "retrospective" study, assessing your behavior from the past based on memory. Now I want you to conduct a "prospective" study where you use the grid below to track your alcohol intake this coming week. If you're out with friends or at a party, you may not want to take your workbook with you, so you can download this chart to carry around with you at http://new harbinger.com/47438 to keep count. You can also use a common method that we teach in a type of treatment called "controlled drinking," where you collect your bottle caps in your pocket. You can keep track by downloading a simple counter app on your phone. Fill in this chart at the end of each day.

Prospective Drinking Chart

Monday	Tuesday	Wednesday	Thursday	Friday	Saturday	Sunday	Total	Average (Total/7)

Memory Strategy: External Memory Aids

One troubling thing I see a lot is that many people don't take drugs that they need to take to protect their brains, like medications for blood pressure and diabetes. This is where the memory strategy of external memory aids comes in handy. Using alarms on your phone or can't-miss reminders, like a sticky note on the coffee pot, can be remarkably effective.

External memory aids make up a group of memory strategies that help you remember by externalizing the information, getting it out of your head. An external memory aid is anything that holds a memory that can be referenced later and can serve as a cue to help trigger a memory. You've been doing a fair amount of externalizing by using the writing step of WOPR, but here are some other strategies.

Buy, Fill, and Use a Pillbox

Using a pillbox does not make you old. It makes you responsible. I recommend that everyone who takes daily medication use a pillbox, regardless of their age. There is a reason birth control pills come in those packs with all the days marked. Even twenty-year-olds forget to take medications, or shall we say especially twenty-year-olds? I wish all medications came that way. Give up resisting the pillbox. Remembering medication is an important memory task to outsource.

When will you buy your pillbox? _____

How often will you fill your pillbox? _____

Use a Calendar

So many people complain about missing appointments, but when I ask if they use a calendar, they often say no. Using a calendar is a habit, and maybe you were proficient at using a calendar at one point in your life, but often when people retire or have a change in responsibilities, calendar use can wane. If you do not already use a calendar to keep up with appointments, visits with friends, and daily tasks, now is the time to start. Here are some tips.

There are lots of different calendars. Many people these days use the calendars on their cell phones. Cell phone calendars are nice because you tend to have your phone with you almost all the time and they have nice alarms and reminders. You can also adjust them to be viewed by day, week, month, or year, and you can share them with your family. But they may not be for everyone, particularly if you're having trouble adjusting to technology or if you need your info out in the open.

The standard one-month calendar that hangs on the wall is great for seeing your appointments out in the open and for referencing them quickly. You may want to use a dry-erase board to put the date really large in your field of view each day so you can keep track that way.

A date book with one week per page or one day per page may be what you need, particularly if you want to use it as a "memory bible" that allows you to improve both your prospective (remembering things in the future) and your retrospective memory (sort of like a diary to help you remember what you did yesterday). Many people with memory loss find this habit of using a calendar/diary ("memory bible") to be very helpful, so they can go back and reference important memories, like birthday parties, lunch with friends, and phone calls to the grandkids.

Let's digest. What sort of calendar do you think will work best for you? If you already use a calendar, are there any tweaks or upgrades you can do to your "calendaring"?

_____

_____

_____

Even if you think that you will remember something, put it on your calendar anyway. It's better to have things on your calendar that you remembered than to forget or to miss an appointment or special event. Also, what good is having something in your calendar if you never look at it? Make it a habit to look at your calendar many times a day, especially first thing in the morning and before you go to bed.

Alarms and Reminders

Even if you are not all that tech savvy, many devices, including your phone, can provide alarms and reminders for things like taking medication, waking up, and checking your blood sugar. Set them, use them, and then use them again. These days, you can even just tell Siri, Alexa, or Google to set your alarms and reminders.

Let's digest. Jot down some ideas you have for new ways you want to "spruce up" your use of calendars and alerts.

_____

_____

_____

The Special Spot

Putting important items in a special spot and being disciplined about keeping them there is another great external memory aid. In the CogSMART program (Twamley et al. 2012), therapists call this a "home" for your things. An important way to improve your memory is to identify a home or special spot for your keys, phone, wallet, calendar, and any daily notebook that you use. A basket near the door that you use most often to come and go is ideal. If you don't have a special spot or a home for your keys, wallet, calendar, and so forth, make one *right now*. I'll wait.

Where is it? (Shhh...I won't tell anyone.) _____

Put the bills you need to pay in a special spot, ideally somewhere visible to you to serve as a visual reminder to pay them. Other less frequently accessed documents should also have a special spot, but it should be more out of the way of your everyday space, like a file drawer. Get some help with organizing this if this is a struggle for you. Where are these places for you?

Bills to pay live here: _____

Documents are filed here: _____

People who can help you organize this stuff include: _____

Can't-Miss Reminders

I really like this strategy from the CogSMART program (Twamley et al. 2012). Can't-miss reminders involve what the name implies: placing a reminder in an obvious place where you can't miss it. For example, you can tape a note to your coffee pot to feed the dog or use a dry-erase marker to write yourself a note on your bathroom mirror to *take your pills*. If you need to take something with you on your next outing, you can hang it from the handle of the door that you use to leave the house.

So, let's not forget that medications are often an essential component of a healthy and optimal memory. It's important to talk frequently with your doctor about ways to improve your memory and any potential side effects that your medications may have on your memory. And what good is a medication if you don't remember to take it? Use external memory aids like a pillbox, calendar, special spot, and alarms to help your memory out, and you will be a memory pro.

Chapter 12

Socialize with Purpose

In our last chapter together, we will focus on rounding out your social life and your sense of purpose as additional ways of improving your memory now and in the long run. Investing in your social life and spiritual well-being can pay big returns as you continue to improve your memory.

How Living with A Sense of Purpose Helps Your Memory

The Rush Memory and Aging Project at Rush University Medical Center in Chicago has contributed heavily to our understanding of the factors that affect brain 401(k) investing. One of the many outcomes of this large-scale, longitudinal (following the same people over the long term) study showed that people who reported having a stronger sense of purpose in their lives had better cognitive reserve. Thus, they better withstood the effects of Alzheimer's disease pathology growing in their brains (Bennett et al. 2012).

There is also growing evidence to suggest that orienting to a sense of purpose can improve your cognitive engagement. This is the extent to which you are focused on what you're doing, maybe even getting lost in your work (Burrow, Agans, and Rainone 2018; Chaudhary 2019). Engagement is crucial for your learning and memory as we have discussed many times in this book, providing much-needed focus. You can't expect to remember what you don't notice, right?

Purpose is your "why," your reason for living, why you do what you do. It can be overwhelming to try to figure out your overall purpose in life. The great thing about purpose is that you don't have to solve that existential puzzle to reap the benefits. One thing you can do is define your purpose moment to moment. Ask yourself: What is my purpose in this moment, this task, this day? Why am I doing it?

Try it. What is your purpose in completing this chapter? Why do you want to read this chapter? What do you hope to gain?

_____

_____

_____

Another way to access your purpose is by asking yourself some of those "deathbed questions," like _What would I regret if I died today?_

_____

_____

_____

_____

Boom. Here's your purpose. Sort of like a bucket list, but better.

Here are a couple of other questions: What was I put here on earth to do? Why do I exist? And before you go getting all hard on yourself, let me just tell you that you exist for a reason. You are a gift. You also get to choose, discern, and decide what that reason is.

A purpose statement can also be aspirational—it may not exactly match your current lifestyle. I wrote a purpose statement for myself recently. It was hard to come up with one on my own, but I found some really great examples in a book called _Beyond Time Management: Business with Purpose_ by Robert Wright (1996). If I had written my purpose statement with my life as I was living it, it would have been something like "I live to work hard, giving freely of myself until I feel drained and resentful," so I tweaked it and made it aspirational. "I live to have fun, enjoying a long and healthy life, maintaining a high standard of living for my own satisfaction so I can make a difference for my family and the world and give back to help those in need." I gotta tell you, this purpose statement is really motivating, and it keeps me on track with my self-care. Often I forget to have fun, enjoy myself, maintain high living standards, and ensure I'm satisfied. This gets in the way of my yearning to make a difference for my family and the world, and how can I ever give back if I'm in a lack and scarcity mind-set all of the time? So take some time to consider your purpose, making sure you're taking care of yourself in the process.

Jot down some ideas about your purpose here:

_____

_____

_____

_____

We began this book by exploring why you want a better memory, and in the physical activity chapter you wrote down your whys for being more physically active. It seems only fitting that we close out the book the same way. Perhaps your why, or your purpose in having a better memory, has changed a bit over the course of the book. This is also a place to go beyond simply having a better memory and reflect on your life's purpose. So let's do the "keep your why close by" exercise again.

Whether it's leaving a legacy for your kids, snowboarding when you're seventy, or making a difference in your career, why do you want to build and maintain a stronger memory? What is your purpose in having a better memory? What is your purpose in life?

_____   _____

_____   _____

_____   _____

_____   _____

_____   _____

Socialization and Memory

Our bodies get unhappy when we don't get our social needs met. Many studies have shown that social isolation, particularly loneliness, is a health risk. Some estimates show that it is as bad for your health as smoking, particularly in terms of how many years it takes off your life (Pantell et al. 2013). Given that what's good for the body is good for the brain, it should come as no surprise that social isolation and loneliness also increase your risk for memory loss and dementia. People who have infrequent social contact and little social activity participation (Kuiper et al. 2015), as well as people who live alone and people who are not in a committed relationship (Sundström, Westerlund, and Kotyrlo 2016), are at much higher risk for all types of dementia.

Being around and interacting with other people may be one of the most efficient forms of brain exercise. I'm willing to wager real money that it's better brain exercise than any brain game around. Just think about it. Even the act of having a simple conversation activates pretty much your whole entire brain. You're listening and learning new things, so the language and memory centers in your temporal lobe are activated. You're processing visual cues from gestures and body language, activating your occipital and parietal lobes. You're pulling up memories, speaking, being nice, waiting your turn, and planning what you want to say, activating your frontal lobes. You're connecting emotionally and processing and regulating emotional cues, activating your amygdala and other brain structures related to empathy and concentration. That's basically your whole entire brain, and that's just a simple conversation. Add to that other things you do with friends, like planning outings together, picking a restaurant, exploring a new part of town, and traveling together, and you can see how being around other people is a really efficient form of brain stimulation. Plus, friends make really great external memory aids, right? They can hold bits of memories that you share together, and reminiscing brings up those old memories for repetition and reencoding.

Even though high-quality relationships are important, evidence shows that your level of satisfaction in your social network actually matters less than the amount of socializing you do. This means that even people who complain about their friends still have a lower risk for dementia than people with few friends (Kuiper et al. 2015). This can actually relieve the pressure a bit, don't you think? Who cares? Get out there and talk to people!

Are You Engaged?

How much do you actually interact with the people in your life? Are you just casually aware of each other because you see each other's notifications on Facebook? When was the last time you really talked? When you are talking, how "in" the conversation are you? Are you distracted by thoughts, like planning your grocery list or thinking about what you want to say next? Are you even making eye contact, or are you scrolling through social media or playing a video game while you're talking?

The level at which you engage in conversations matters. If you're only half there, then you've cut out many of the brain benefits listed above, plus you're missing out on a lot of the richness that comes from interacting with other people. That's why the following chart asks you to track your level of engagement as you're tracking your conversations this coming week.

How Frequently Do You Have Conversations?

Track your conversations over the next week.

	Monday	Tuesday	Wednesday	Thursday	Friday	Saturday	Sunday
People I had conversations with (if too many to list, then enter the number of conversations you had)							
How much I felt supported by my relationships (1 is least supported, 10 is most supported)							
The overall quality of my interactions (1 is most negative, 10 is most positive)							
My level of engagement in the conversations (1 is completely zoned-out, 10 is fully engaged and connected to my feelings and the other person's feelings)							

(A downloadable copy of this worksheet is available at http://newharbinger.com/47438.)

Social Support as a Stress Buffer

Another advantage of socialization is that it is a stress buffer. As you learned in chapter 8, acute stress in the moment can rob you of your focus and thereby your memory via limbic or amygdala hijacking, and chronic stress kills off the brain cells you have and prevents you from growing new neurons, aka liming your brain 401(k) investing.

As we evolved into humans, our brains developed this new fancy cortex that gives us our uniquely human abilities, like our language and math skills. But underneath this fancy cortex, we are still social primates, which means that we need each other to survive and thrive, just like a band of gorillas.

In the animal kingdom, we humans are total weaklings. Our teeth really aren't that sharp. We don't have serious claws or big shells on our backs to protect us from predators. Our vision and hearing are subpar compared to other species. In addition to remembering the things that can kill us, in order to survive, we have also had to work together. Our ancestors formed clans and tribes, shared and traded resources, and protected one another. Getting kicked out of the tribe in the early days meant almost certain death. Even though nowadays we have more solid structures and more convenient ways of gathering resources, to survive we still need other humans.

Who You Gonna Call?

List people in your life whom you can call or turn to when something is bothering you. Be creative here. Be sure to include counselors and support lines:

_____   _____

_____   _____

_____   _____

_____   _____

_____   _____

Hopefully you have a better sense of how purpose and socializing can build and support your memory now and as you age. Not only have both of these skills helped me to feel more focused and engaged, but they've brought a lot of fun and enjoyment to my life. I hope you find the same to be true.

Go Forth with a Better Memory

So we made it through all of the neuroscience and the skills. It has absolutely been my pleasure to accompany you on this journey. Thank you for letting me be your guide. I wish you many more years of brain health and confidence in your memory. This may be the end of the book, but I don't consider it to be the end of our work together. Building and maintaining a healthy memory takes daily practice over a lifetime, so feel free to come back from time to time to brush up on your skills. Don't forget to download any worksheets that you may need to support you on your journey at http://newharbinger .com/47438. Stay in touch with me, and I hope we meet again someday.

Acknowledgments

My amazing husband Mike All is the best. He gave me this great last name. He never criticizes my ideas, graciously parents our four daughters as I travel and write, and loves to vacuum, ya'll. He also helped me immensely with the images for this book. My potential is so enhanced by having so much support at home.

Many thanks go to my writing team. To Wendy Millstein at New Harbinger who "found me"; my agent Amy Bishop at Dystel, Goderich & Bourret, LLC, for having my back and giving consistent fangirl feedback; to Jennye Garibaldi, Caleb Beckwith, and Gretel Hakanson at New Harbinger for wonderful editorial guidance. To Ryan Bartholomew at PESI, who helped me "get out there." To my girlfriends for listening and supporting me; you know who you are, plus special thanks to Suzanne Dunne, Kate Dunkley, Karen Young, Sara Barrett, Polina Reyngold, Leanne Searight, and Starla Sholl. To all of the amazing folks in my Women Belong Networking circle, the Wright Foundation for the Realization of Human Potential, and the Inspiring Victory Writing Group. Special thanks to Sarah Victory who was the first person able to communicate to me that I could do this, and Suzanne Nance for her editorial guidance. I also want to acknowledge my amazing staff at the Chicago Center for Cognitive Wellness: Lydia Wardin, PsyD; Steven Bernfeld, PhD; Genevieve Wolff, MA; Martha Tierney, LCSW; Tina Mavalankar, LCSW; Anna Reidy; and Zoë Grubbs, who do their jobs with dedication so I can indulge my passions. My heart is full.

References

Alzheimer's Association. 2009. *Know the 10 Signs: Early Detection Matters.* TS-0066.

American Psychiatric Association. 2013. *Diagnostic and Statistical Manual of Mental Disorders,* 5th ed. Washington, DC: American Psychiatric Association.

Andrade, C., and N. S. Kumar Rao. 2010. "How Antidepressant Drugs Act: A Primer on Neuroplasticity as the Eventual Mediator of Antidepressant Efficacy." *Indian Journal of Psychiatry* 52: 378–386.

Artero, S., M. L. Ancelin, F. Portet, A. Dupuy, C. Berr, J. F. Dartigues, C. Tzourio, O. Rouaud, M. Poncet, F. Pasquier, S. Auriacombe, J. Touchon, and K. Ritchie. 2008. "Risk Profiles for Mild Cognitive Impairment and Progression to Dementia Are Gender Specific." *Journal of Neurology, Neurosurgery, and Psychiatry* 79, no. 9: 979–984.

Asken, B. M., M. J. Sullan, S. T. DeKosky, M. S. Jaffee, and R. M. Bauer. 2017. "Research Gaps and Controversies in Chronic Traumatic Encephalopathy." *JAMA Neurology* 74, no. 10: 1255–1262.

Baddeley, A. 2010. "Working Memory." *Current Biology* 20, no. 4: R136–R140.

Bennett, D. A., J. A. Schneider, A. S. Buchman, L. L. Barnes, P. A. Boyle, and R. S. Wilson. 2012. "Overview and Findings from the Rush Memory and Aging Project." *Current Alzheimer Research* 9, no. 6: 646–663.

Bhattacharyya, K. B. 2017. "James Wenceslaus Papez, His Circuit, and Emotion." *Annals of Indian Academy of Neurology* 20, no. 3: 207–210.

Bolte Taylor, J. 2006. *My Stroke of Insight: A Brain Scientist's Personal Journey.* New York: Viking Press.

Bookheimer, S. 2002. "Functional MRI of Language: New Approaches to Understanding the Cortical Organization of Semantic Processing." *Annual Review of Neuroscience* 25: 151–188.

Brandt, J., A. Buchholz, B. Henry-Barron, D. Vizthum, D. Avramopoulos, and M. C. Cervenka. 2019. "Preliminary Report on the Feasibility and Efficacy of the Modified Atkins Diet for Treatment of Mild Cognitive Impairment and Early Alzheimer's Disease." *Journal of Alzheimer's Disease* 68, no. 3: 969–981.

Burkhardt, T., D. Lüdecke, L. Spies, L. Wittmann, M. Westphal, and J. Flitsch. 2015. "Hippocampal and Cerebellar Atrophy in Patients with Cushing's Disease." *Neurosurgical Focus* 39, no. 5: E5.

Burrow, A. L., J. P. Agans, and N. Rainone. 2018. "Exploring Purpose as a Resource for Promoting Youth Program Engagement." *Journal of Youth Development* 13, no. 4: 164–178.

Cameron, H. A., and E. Gould. 1994. "Adult Neurogenesis Is Regulated by Adrenal Steroids in the Dentate Gyrus." *Neuroscience* 61, no. 2: 203–209.

Chaudhary, R. 2019. "Corporate Social Responsibility Perceptions and Employee Engagement: Role of Psychological Meaningfulness, Safety, and Availability." *Corporate Governance* 19, no. 4: 631–647.

Church, M. K., and D. S. Church. 2013. "Pharmacology of Antihistamines." *Indian Journal of Dermatology* 58, no. 3: 219–224.

Cicerone K. D., D. M. Langenbahn, C. Braden, J. F. Malec, K. Kalmar, M. Fraas, T. Felicetti, L. Laatsch, J. P. Harley, T. Bergquist, J. Azulay, J. Cantor, and T. Ashman. 2011. "Evidence-Based Cognitive Rehabilitation: Updated Review of the Literature from 2003 Through 2008." *Archives of Physical Medicine and Rehabilitation* 92, no. 4: 519–530.

Corballis, M. C. 2014. "Left Brain, Right Brain: Facts and Fantasies." *PLOS Biology* 12, no. 1: e1001767.

Cummings, J. L. 1993. "Frontal-Subcortical Circuits and Human Behavior." *Archives of Neurology* 50, no. 8: 873–880.

Dale, A., and E. Halgren. 2001. "Spatiotemporal Mapping of Brain Activity by Integration of Multiple Imaging Modalities." *Current Opinion in Neurobiology* 11, no. 2: 202–208.

Del Cerro, S., M. Jung, and G. Lynch. 1992. "Benzodiazepines Block Long-Term Potentiation in Slices of Hippocampus and Piriform Cortex." *Neuroscience* 49, no. 1: 1–6.

De Vivo, L., M. Bellesi, W. Marhsall, E. A. Bushong, M. H. Ellisman, G. Tononi, and C. Cirelli. 2017. "Ultrastructural Evidence for Synaptic Scaling Across the Wake/Sleep Cycle." *Science* 355: 507–510.

Doidge, N. 2007. *The Brain That Changes Itself: Stories of Personal Triumph from the Frontiers of Brain Science.* Melbourne, Victoria, Australia: Scribe Publications.

Doyon, J., and H. Benali. 2005. "Reorganization and Plasticity in the Adult Brain During Learning of Motor Skills." *Current Opinion in Neurobiology* 15, no. 2: 161–167.

Engvig, A., A. M. Fjell, L. T. Westlye, T. Moberget, Ø. Sundseth, V. A. Larsen, and K. B. Walhovd. 2012. "Memory Training Impacts Short-Term Changes in Aging White Matter: A Longitudinal Diffusion Tensor Imaging Study." *Human Brain Mapping* 33, no. 10: 2390–2406.

Erickson, K. I., R. L. Leckie, and A. M. Weinstein. 2014. "Physical Activity, Fitness, and Gray Matter Volume." *Neurobiology of Aging,* supplement 2: S20–S28.

Erickson, K. I., C. A. Raji, O. L. Lopez, J. T. Becker, C. Rosano, A. B. Newman, H. M. Gach, P. M. Thompson, A. J. Ho, and L. H. Kuller. 2010. "Physical Activity Predicts Gray Matter Volume in Late Adulthood: The Cardiovascular Health Study." *Neurology* 75, no. 16: 1415–1422.

Erickson, K. I., M. W. Voss, R. S. Prakash, C. Basak, A. Szabo, L. Chaddock, J. S. Kim, S. Heo, H. Alves, S. M. White, T. R. Wojcicki, E. Mailey, V. J. Vieira, S. A. Martin, B. D. Pence, J. A. Woods, E. McAuley, and A. F. Kramer. 2011. "Exercise Training Increases Size of Hippocampus and Improves Memory." *Proceedings of the National Academy of Sciences* 108, no. 7: 3017–3022.

Eriksson, P. S., E. Perfilieva, T. Björk-Eriksson, A. Alborn, C. Noardborg, D. A. Peterson, and F. H. Gage. 1998. "Neurogenesis in the Adult Human Hippocampus." *Nature Medicine* 4: 1313–1317.

Fama, R., and E. V. Sullivan. 2015. "Thalamic Structures and Associated Cognitive Functions: Relations with Age and Aging." *Neuroscience & Biobehavioral Reviews* 54: 29–37.

Fernandez, A., and E. Goldberg. 2009. *The SharpBrains Guide to Brain Fitness.* San Francisco: SharpBrains, Inc.

Gladwell, M. 2008. *Outliers: The Story of Success.* New York: Little, Brown, and Company.

Goldman-Rakic, P. S. 1995. "Cellular Basis of Working Memory." *Neuron* 14: 477–485.

Goleman, D. 1995. *Emotional Intelligence: Why It Can Matter More Than IQ.* New York: Bantam Books.

Gould E., P. Tanapat, T. Rydel, and N. Hastings. 2000. "Regulation of Hippocampal Neurogenesis in Adulthood." *Biological Psychiatry* 48, no. 8: 715–720.

Gradari, S., A. Pallé, K. R. McGreevy, Á. Fontán-Lozano, and J. L. Trejo. 2016. "Can Exercise Make You Smarter, Happier, and Have More Neurons? A Hermetic Perspective." *Frontiers in Neuroscience* 10: 93.

Han, K., S. B. Chapman, and D. C. Krawczyk. 2018. "Neuroplasticity of Cognitive Control Networks Following Cognitive Training for Chronic Traumatic Brain Injury." *NeuroImage* 18: 262–278.

Hanson, R. 2009. *Buddha's Brain: The Practical Neuroscience of Happiness, Love, and Wisdom.* Oakland, CA: New Harbinger Publications.

Harbishettar, V., P. K. Pal, Y. C. J. Reddy, and K. Thennarasu. 2005. "Is There a Relationship Between Parkinson's Disease and Obsessive Compulsive Disorder?" *Parkinsonism & Related Disorders* 11, no. 2: 85–88.

Herbert, L. E., J. Weuve, P. A. Scherr, and D. A. Evans. 2013. "Alzheimer Disease in the United States (2010–2050) Estimated Using the 2010 Census." *Neurology* 80, no. 19: 1778–1783.

Huntley J. D., A. Hampshire, D. Bor, A. Owen, and R. J. Howard. 2017. "Adaptive Working Memory Strategy Training in Early Alzheimer's Disease: Randomized Controlled Trial." *British Journal of Psychiatry* 210, no. 1: 61–66.

Imbimbo, B. P., J. Lombard, and N. Pomara, N. 2005. "Pathophysiology of Alzheimer's Disease." *Neuroimaging Clinics of North America* 15, no. 4: 727–753.

Jessen, N. A., A. S. Finmann Munk, I. Lundgaard, and M. Nedergaard. 2015. "The Glymphatic System: A Beginner's Guide." *Neurochemical Research* 40, no. 12: 2583–2599.

Kabat-Zinn, J. 1994. *Wherever You Go, There You Are: Mindfulness Meditation in Everyday Life.* New York: Hyperion Press.

Katzman, R., M. Aronson, P. Flud, C. Kawas, T. Brown, H. Morgenstern, W. Frishman, L. Gidez, H. Eder, and W. L. Ooi. 1989. "Development of Dementing Illnesses in an 80-Year-Old Volunteer Cohort." *Annals of Neurology* 25, no. 4: 317–324.

Kavirajan. H., and L. S. Schneider. 2007. "Efficacy and Adverse Effects of Cholinesterase Inhibitors and Memantine in Vascular Dementia: A Meta-Analysis of Randomised Controlled Trials." *Lancet Neurology* 6, no. 9: 782–792.

Kelley, M., B. Ulin, and L. C. McGuire. 2018. "Reducing the Risk of Alzheimer's Disease and Maintaining Brain Health in an Aging Society." *Public Health Reports* 133, no. 3: 225–229.

Kuiper, J. S., M. Zuidersma, R. C. Oude Voshaar, S. U. Zuidema, E. R. van den Heuvel, R. P. Stolk, and N. Smidt. 2015. "Social Relationships and Risk of Dementia: A Systematic Review and Meta-Analysis of Longitudinal Cohort Studies." *Ageing Research Reviews* 22: 39–57.

Langer, E. 2014. "Science of Mindlessness and Mindfulness." Podcast. *On Being with Krista Tippett* (May 29), https://onbeing.org/programs/ellen-langer-science-of-mindlessness-and-mindfulness-nov2017/.

LeDoux, J. 2012. "Rethinking the Emotional Brain." *Neuron* 73, no. 4: 653–676.

Livingston, G., A. Sommerlad, V. Orgeta, S. G. Costafreda, J. Huntley, D. Ames, et al. 2017. "Dementia Prevention, Intervention, and Care." *The Lancet Commissions* 390: 2673–2734.

Loftus, E. F. 2005. "Planting Misinformation in the Human Mind: A 30-Year Investigation of the Malleability of Memory." *Learning and Memory* 12: 361–366.

Martínez-Lapiscina, E. H., P. Clavero, E. Toledo, R. Estruch, J. Salas-Salvado, B. San Julian, A. Sanchez-Tainta, E. Ros, C. Valls-Pedret, and M. Á. Martinez-Gonzalez. 2013. "Mediterranean Diet Improves Cognition: The PREDIMED-NAVARRA Randomized Trial." *Journal of Neurology, Neurosurgery, and Psychiatry* 84: 1318–1325.

Marx, P. 2013. "Mentally Fit: Workouts at the Brain Gym." *New Yorker*, July 29, 24–37.

McCarley, R. W. 2007. "Neurobiology of REM and NREM Sleep." *Sleep Medicine* 8, no. 4: 302–330.

McGonigal, K. 2015. *The Upside of Stress: Why Stress is Good for You, and How to Get Good at It.* New York: Avery Publishing.

Merzenich, M. M., R. J. Nelson, M. P. Stryker, M. S. Cynader, A. Schoppmann, and J. M. Zook. 1984. "Somatosensory Cortical Map Changes Following Digit Amputation in Adult Monkeys." *The Journal of Comparative Neurology* 224: 591–605.

Mitchell, A. J., and M. Shiri-Feshki. 2009. "Rate of Progression of Mild Cognitive Impairment to Dementia—Meta-Analysis of 41 Robust Inception Cohort Studies." *Acta Psychiatrica Scandinavica* 119, no. 4: 252–265.

Mitchell, J. T., L. Zylowska, and S. H. Kollins. 2015. "Mindfulness Meditation Training for Attention Deficit/Hyperactivity Disorder in Adulthood: Current Empirical Support, Treatment Overview, and Future Directions." *Cognitive Behavioral Practice* 22, no. 2: 172–191.

Morris, M. C., J. Brockman, J. A. Schneider, Y. Wang, D. A. Bennett, C. C. Tangney, and O. van de Rest. 2016. "Association of Seafood Consumption, Brain Mercury Level, and APOE ε4 Status with Brain Neuropathology in Older Adults." *Journal of the American Medical Association* 315, no. 5: 489–497.

Morris, M. C., C. C. Tangney, Y. Wang, F. M. Sacks, L. L. Barnes, D. A. Bennett, and N. T. Aggarwal. 2015. "MIND Diet Slows Cognitive Decline with Aging." *Alzheimer's & Dementia* 11, no. 9: 1015–1022.

Moyer, C. A., S. S. Sonnad, S. L. Garetz, J. I. Helman, and R. D. Chervin. 2001. "Quality of Life in Obstructive Sleep Apnea: A Systematic Review of the Literature." *Sleep Medicine* 2, no. 6: 477–491.

Neth, B. J., J. Graff-Radford, M. M. Mielke, S. A. Przybelski, T. G. Lesnick, C. G. Schwarz, R. I. Reid, M. L. Senjem, V. J. Lowe, M. M. Machulda, R. C. Petersen, C. R. Jack, Jr., D. S. Knopman, and P. Vemuri. 2020. "Relationship Between Risk Factors and Brain Reserve in Late Middle Age: Implications for Cognitive Aging." *Frontiers in Aging Neuroscience* 11: 1–11.

Nicoll, R. A. 2017. "A Brief History of Long-Term Potentiation." *Neuron* 9, no. 23: 281–290.

Niendam, T. A., A. R. Laird, K. L. Ray, Y. M. Dean, D. C. Glahn, and C. S. Carter. 2012. "Meta-Analytic Evidence for a Superordinate Cognitive Control Network Subserving Diverse Executive Functions." *Cognitive Affective & Behavioral Neuroscience* 12, no. 2: 241–268.

Pantell, M., D. Rehkopf, D. Jutte, S. L. Syme, J. Balmes, and N. Adler. 2013. "Social Isolation: A Predictor of Mortality Comparable to Traditional Clinical Risk Factors." *American Journal of Public Health* 103, no. 11: 2056–2062.

Phua, C. S., L. Jayaram, and T. Wijeratne. 2017. "Relationship Between Sleep Duration and Risk Factors for Stroke." *Frontiers in Neurology* 8: 1–6.

Pittman, C. M., and E. M. Karle. 2015. *Rewire Your Anxious Brain: How to Use the Neuroscience of Fear to End Anxiety, Panic, and Worry.* Oakland, CA: New Harbinger Publications.

Poldrack, R. A., J. Clark, E. J. Pare-Blagoev, D. Shohamy, J. Creso Moyano, C. Myers, and M. A. Gluck. 2001. "Interactive Memory Systems in the Human Brain." *Nature* 414: 546–550.

Raichle, M. E., A. M. MacLeod, A. Z. Snyder, W. J. Powers, D. A. Gusnard, and G. L. Shulman. 2001. "A Default Mode of Brain Function." *Proceedings of the National Academy of Sciences* 98, no. 2: 676–682.

Rink, C., and S. Khanna. 2011. "Significance of Brain Tissue Oxygenation and the Arachidonic Acid Cascade in Stroke." *Antioxidants & Redox Signaling* 14, no. 10: 1889–1903.

Sabia, S., A. Fayosse, J. Dumurgier, A. Dugrovot, T. Akbaraly, A. Britton, M. Kivimäki, and A. Singh-Manoux. 2018. "Alcohol Consumption and Risk for Dementia: 23 Year Follow-Up of Whitehall II Cohort Study." *BMJ* 362: k2927.

Sacks, F. M., L. J. Appel, T. J. Moore, E. Obarzanek, W. M. Vollmer, L. P. Svetkey, G. A. Bray, T. M. Vogt,
J. A. Cutler, M. M. Windhauser, P. H. Lin, and N. Karanja. 1999. "A Dietary Approach to Prevent Hypertension: A Review of the Dietary Approaches to Stop Hypertension (DASH) Study." *Clinical Cardiology* 22: III6–10.

Sadato, N., A. Pascual-Leone, J. Grafman, V. Ibañez, M. P. Deiber, G. Dold, and M. Hallett. 1996. "Activation of the Primary Visual Cortex by Braille Reading in Blind Subjects." *Nature* 380: 526–528.

Salthouse, T. A. 2009. "When Does Age-Related Cognitive Decline Begin?" *Neurobiology of Aging* 30: 507–514.

Sapolsky, R. M. 2004. *Why Zebras Don't Get Ulcers*, 3rd ed. New York: Holt Paperbacks.

Savić, M. M., D. I. Obradović, N. D. Ugrešić, and D. R. Boknjić. 2005. "Memory Effects of Benzodiazepines: Memory Stages and Types Versus Binding-Site Subtypes." *Neural Plasticity* 12, no. 4: 289–298.

Schacter, D. L., D. R. Addis, D. Hassabis, V. C. Martin, R. N. Spreng, and K. K. Szpunar. 2012. "The Future of Memory: Remembering, Imagining, and the Brain." *Neuron* 76, no. 4: 677–694.

Siegel, J. M. 2001. "The REM Sleep-Memory Consolidation Hypothesis." *Science* 294: 1058–1063.

Sng, E., E. Frith, and P. D. Loprinzi. 2018. "Temporal Effects of Acute Walking Exercise on Learning and Memory Function." *American Journal of Health Promotion* 32, no. 7: 1518–1525.

Socci, V., D. Tempesta, G. Desideri, L. De Gennaro, and M. Ferrara. 2017. "Enhancing Human Cognition with Cocoa Flavonoids." *Frontiers in Nutrition* 4: 1–7.

Squire, L. R. 2009. "The Legacy of Patient H. M. for Neuroscience." *Neuron* 61, no. 1: 6–9.

Stern, Y. 2002. "What Is Cognitive Reserve? Theory and Research Applications of the Reserve Concept." *Journal of the International Neuropsychological Society* 8: 448–460.

Stringer, A. Y. 2007a. *Ecologically Oriented Neurorehabilitation of Memory*. Los Angeles: Western Psychological Services.

Stringer, A. Y. 2007b. "Ecologically Oriented Neurorehabilitation of Memory: Robustness of Outcome Across Diagnosis and Severity." *Brain Injury* 25, no. 2: 169–178.

Sundström, A., O. Westerlund, and E. Kotyrlo. 2016. "Marital Status and Risk of Dementia: A Nationwide Population-Based Prospective Study from Sweden." *British Medical Journal Open* 6, no. 1: e008565.

Taren, A. A., J. D. Creswell, and P. J. Gianaros. 2013. "Dispositional Mindfulness Co-Varies with Smaller Amygdala and Caudate Volumes in Community Adults." *PLOS One* 8: 1–7.

Trichopoulou, A., T. Costacou, C. Bamia, and D. Trichopoulos. 2003. "Adherence to a Mediterranean Diet and Survival in a Greek Population." *New England Journal of Medicine* 348, no. 26: 2599–2608.

Twamley, E., M. Huckans, S-M. Tun, L. Hutson, S. Noonan, G. Savla, A. Jak, D. Schiehser, and D. Storzbach. 2012. *Compensatory Cognitive Training for Traumatic Brain Injury: Facilitator's Guide*. http://www.cogsmart.com/resources.

Underwood, E. 2016. "Brain Game-Maker Fined $2 Million for Lumosity False Advertising." *Science*, January 5. https://www.sciencemag.org/news/2016/01/brain-game-maker-fined-2-million-lumosity-false-advertising

Van der Helm, E., J. Yao, S. Dutt, V. Rao, J. M. Salentin, and M. P. Walker. 2011. "REM Sleep Depotentiates Amygdala Activity to Previous Emotional Experiences." *Current Biology* 21, no. 23: 2029–2032.

Van de Rest, O., Y. Wang, L. L. Barnes, C. Tangney, D. A. Bennett, and M. C. Morris. 2016. "APOE ε4 and the Associations of Seafood and Long-Chain Omega-3 Fatty Acids with Cognitive Decline." *Neurology* 86, no. 22: 2063–2070.

Vitanova, K. S., K. M. Stringer, D. P. Benitez, J. Brenton, and D. M. Cummings. 2019. "Dementia Associated with Disorders of the Basal Ganglia." *Journal of Neuroscience Research* 97. https://doi.org/10.1002/jnr.24508.

White, E. J., S. A. Hutka, L. J. Williams, and S. Moreno. 2013. "Learning, Neural Plasticity and Sensitive Periods: Implications for Language Acquisition, Music Training and Transfer Across the Lifespan." *Frontiers in Systems Neuroscience* 7: 1–18.

Williamson, A., and A. Feyer. 2000. "Moderate Sleep Deprivation Produces Impairments in Cognitive and Motor Performance Equivalent to Legally Prescribed Levels of Alcohol Intoxication." *Occupational and Environmental Medicine* 57, no. 10: 649–655.

Winer, J. R., B. A. Mander, R. F. Helfrich, A. Maass, T. M. Harrison, S. L. Baker, R. T. Knight, W. J. Jagust, and M. P. Walker. 2019. "Sleep as a Potential Biomarker of Tau and β-Amyloid Burden in the Human Brain." *The Journal of Neuroscience* 39, no 32: 6315–6324.

Wise, S. P. 1996. "The Role of the Basal Ganglia in Procedural Memory." *Seminars in Neuroscience* 8, no. 1: 39–46.

Woolett, K., and E. A. Maguire. 2011. "Acquiring 'the Knowledge' of London's Layout Drives Structural Brain Changes." *Current Biology* 21: 2109–2114.

Wright, R. J. 1996. *Beyond Time Management: Business with Purpose.* Newton, MA: Butterworth-Heinemann.

Zeidan, F., S. K. Johnson, B. J. Diamond, Z. David, and P. Goolkasian. 2010. "Mindfulness Meditation Improves Cognition: Evidence of Brief Mental Training." *Consciousness and Cognition* 19: 597–605.

Zimprich, D., P. Rast, and M. Martin. 2008. "Individual Differences in Verbal Learning in Old Age." In *Handbook of Cognitive Aging: Interdisciplinary Perspectives,* edited by S. M. Hoffer and D. F. Alwin. Thousand Oaks, CA: Sage Publications, Inc.

Sherrie D. All, PhD, is passionate about empowering people to use their brains brilliantly to live better, lead better, and love better. She is an international speaker; writer; licensed clinical neurore-habilitation psychologist; brain health expert; and owner and director of the Chicago Center for Cognitive Wellness—a private group practice dedicated to helping people with anxiety, depression, and physical symptoms, with a particular focus on helping adults experiencing cognitive decline through assessment and treatment services. As a trained neuropsychologist, Sherrie brings her detailed understanding of the brain to uniquely address the needs of people with traumatic brain injury (TBI), multiple sclerosis (MS), dementia, and more.

Foreword writer **Paul E. Bendheim, MD**, is clinical professor of neurology at the University of Arizona College of Medicine; founder and chief medical officer of BrainSavers®; and author of *The Brain Training Revolution*.

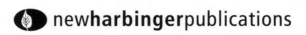

MORE BOOKS from
NEW HARBINGER PUBLICATIONS

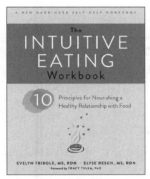
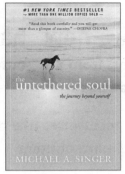
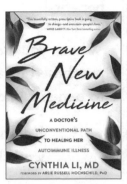
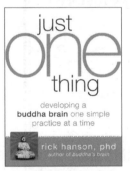
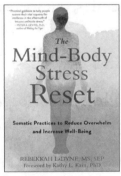
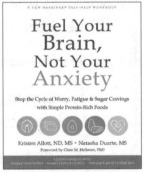

Register your **new harbinger** titles for additional benefits!

When you register your **new harbinger** title—purchased in any format, from any source—you get access to benefits like the following:

- Downloadable accessories like printable worksheets and extra content

- Instructional videos and audio files

- Information about updates, corrections, and new editions

Not every title has accessories, but we're adding new material all the time.

Access free accessories in 3 easy steps:

1. Sign in at NewHarbinger.com (or **register** to create an account).

2. Click on **register a book**. Search for your title and click the **register** button when it appears.

3. Click on the **book cover or title** to go to its details page. Click on **accessories** to view and access files.

That's all there is to it!

If you need help, visit:

NewHarbinger.com/accessories

new harbinger
CELEBRATING
40 YEARS